AF703973

DEFAMED

DEFAMED

How Physicians Pursue Justice:
A Primer for Unjustified Legal Actions
Against Innocent Practitioners

Copyright © 2025

Print ISBN: 979-8-9917852-0-4

Ebook ISBN:979-8-9917852-1-1

Disclaimers:

This is a work of fiction gathering experiences from several physicians in a fictitious manner. Any names, places, or details are not intended and do not portray actual persons institutions or events.

This work does not provide legal advice. The author is not an attorney. Please consult with an attorney for any legal advice.

TABLE OF CONTENTS

INTRODUCTION

Dr. Fuentes, a successful and famous interventional cardiologist, was abruptly suspended—discovering the hard way that you can be removed from your position, titles, and functions at any moment without immediate remedy. He found himself at the mercy of the full power of hospital administrations, nurse unions, and competing physicians on the medical executive committees. He faced retaliation from the hospital's legal team when he attempted to exercise his right for a hearing, getting drawn into a seemingly endless process aimed to destroy him financially and mentally. And his life was put on pause for three years, with no end in sight.

But—he learned to face this challenging situation in a true trial by fire.

What is covered in this book is not taught in medical schools, and yet it can affect the life and career of any practitioner. *Defamed* is written with the intention to help physicians, attorneys, and health care administrators deal with the complex issues surrounding a physician's unfair revocation or suspension of privileges.

I hope you never face such unjustified legal action, but should any occur, then perhaps the story of Dr. Fuentes and this primer of what happened can aid you on your own quest for justice.

THE KEY PLAYERS

Dr. Manuel Fuentes: Chief of Interventional cardiology

Mr. Alan Rogers, Attorney to Dr. Fuentes —supportive

Dr. Anabella Strong, Partner of Dr. Fuentes —supportive

Dr. Bruce Waine, Partner of Dr. Fuentes —supportive

Dr. Scott Summers, Partner of Dr. Fuentes —supportive

Dr. Robert Grant: Chief of cardiology —supportive

Dr. Ludovic Friedland: chairman of medicine —supportive

Dr. Rafael Navin, Ex CMO —neutral

Jane Clark, RN, cath lab nurse —neutral

Dr. Natasha Romanov, key witness against Dr. Brauer —supportive

Dr. Romeo Sabatini, anesthesiologist —supportive

Carmel Asuncion, physician assistant for interventional: cardiology —supportive

Sam Santori, cath lab technician —supportive

Miguel de Guerra, cath lab technician —supportive

The Antagonists

Mr. Dick Kosakov, attorney for the hospital

Mrs. Clara Harari, director of personnel, HR

Mr. Alan Troy, HR representative

Dr. Mary Rattner, medical staff president

Dr. Georges Livingstone, CMO Phoenix Hospital

Mrs. Laura Browning, CEO Phoenix Hospital

Mr. Ethan Sims, director of medical administration

Dr. Christina Taley: Chair of surgery

Dr. Marc Reely, general surgeon, mediator between cardiothoracic and interventional cardiology

Dr. Janet Brauer: cardiothoracic surgeon

Dr. Ralph Liota cardiothoracic surgeon

Dr. Samantha Klein, hospitalist

Dr. Stephanie Balley, member of the investigative committee

Nurse Olivia Grogun, union rep

Nurse Patrick Noah, coronary care unit nurse

Nurse Marc McDonough, medicine floor nurse

Nurse Georgina Lark, cath lab nurse

Robert Blevins, RN, nurse director of the cath lab

Christopher Simonar, RN, nurse manager of the cath lab

Lara Malcom, VP operation

CHAPTER 1

THE SUSPENSION

On a typical Thursday afternoon, Dr. Manuel Fuentes was in the midst of a busy day in the cath lab. He had already performed three cases and had another four cases scheduled, two of them complex and the other two pretty straight forward. He was moving steadily with good support from anesthesia and his assistants.

Dr. Fuentes, an internationally renowned interventional cardiologist, is the chief of the coronary unit at a large academic hospital in the Phoenix metro area. He was hired six years ago to create an advanced cardiology program and had fulfilled his promises. In just under five years, he had indeed increased the volume of procedures by 175 percent, creating an elite service in the region encompassing a service line with three other interventional cardiologists (Dr. Anabella Strong, Dr. Bruce Waine, and Dr. Scott Summers), two physician assistants, two advanced instructors, two XR technicians and several dedicated nurses and nurse practitioners.

That said, Dr. Fuentes noticed there could be further improvement. In particular, he wondered—*could they more efficiently serve patients?*

A few weeks prior, Dr. Fuentes, in an attempt to improve cost effectiveness of the cath lab, hired two medical students, on summer break from the university of Arizona, to run a turnover project. By placing them at the door of procedure rooms and having them capture the real turnover time – independently from any information entered in the computer by the nurses – he was able to establish five interesting facts:

1. Some nurses were resetting the timer capturing room cleaning time, intentionally delaying the next case.
2. Some nurses were delaying starting the timer of the room while cleaning was happening.
3. Transportation for inpatients was not always called early enough, resulting in delaying the arrival of the patient in the unit.
4. After 4 PM, there was a clear slowing of all nursing operations with the intent to reach 5 PM, at which time two rooms out of four closed in the cath lab.
5. Patients are noted to remain much longer in the room than what was captured in the computer.

At the conclusion of this project, he intended to present his findings to the hospital leadership. Dr. Fuentes never realized that this project would be one of the key reasons behind his demise.

The Fateful Day

In the early afternoon, Dr. Fuentes was in his office finishing charting a procedure before starting the next one. The hospital's chairman of medicine, Dr. Ludovic Friedland, along with his administrative assistant, suddenly entered into Dr. Fuentes's office and asked him to come with him for an emergency meeting at once.

Dr. Fuentes was surprised by this visit. Indeed, the chairman of medicine never came to the cardiology suite—and never anywhere unannounced. Since he was about to start another procedure, he asked if they could meet near the cath lab, but the chair insisted that this meeting needed to happen immediately and privately in his office.

Dr. Fuentes left the unit after letting one of his unit nurses know that the next case likely will be delayed. He also asked her to apologize on his behalf to the patients for this unexpected delay.

He reached the medical school building where the chairman of medicine office was located. He entered the chairman's office and was asked to sit on a chair across from the chairman's desk.

There the chairman announced to Dr. Fuentes that he was put in "precautionary suspension" effective immediately.

Manuel was stunned. He never imagined hearing those words. He asked why and was told that a concerning complaints had come from Human Resources (HR), which led to the personnel director (Clara Harari) to request precautionary suspension from the medical staff president (Dr. Mary Rattner) and the chief medical officer (Dr. Georges Livingstone).

Chairman Dr. Ludovic Friedland told Dr. Fuentes that he tried his best to stop the suspension, but leadership of the hospital was very determined in imposing it.

He was asked to leave the facility at once or he could be escorted out by security. After more than twenty years in a career without a single significant incident within any institution, Dr. Fuentes found himself leaving the hospital to avoid the shame of being escorted out.

"Guilty" Until Proven Innocent

PRECAUTIONARY SUSPENSION means the imposition of an immediate suspension or restriction of clinical privileges, based on concerns that the failure to do so may result in imminent danger to the health and/or safety of any individual or the organization.[1]

The key feature of a precautionary suspension is the concept of an imminent danger justifying this action.

Typically, in most hospitals a suspension requires the approval of two of the following individuals: chief medical officer, chief operating officer, president of medical staff office and/or chief of service of the respective physician concerned (Medicine for a cardiologist, Surgery for a laparoscopic surgeon).

In reality, there is no major difference between different types of suspensions, ***whether called immediate, summary, emergency, or precautionary****. The timeline is really the key here and needs to be understood very clearly by the physician.*

---

1 Wermuth HR, Sergent SR. The National Practitioner Data Bank. 2023 May 1. In: StatPearls [Internet]. Treasure Island (FL): StatPearls Publishing; 2023 Jan–. PMID: 32644634. Pubmed

The National Practitioner Data Bank (NPDB) views suspensions in a time-based manner: ***any suspension in effect for more than 30 days before an action is taken by an authorized hospital committee or body, must be reported to the NPDB.***[2]

If the authorized hospital committee or body does not confirm the initial action or takes a different professional review action, a Revision-to-Action Report must be submitted. If the authorized hospital committee or body vacates the summary suspension, the entity must void the previous report submitted to the NPDB (see below).[3]

Indeed, a precautionary or temporary suspension is typically reviewed and confirmed by a hospital committee, such as a medical executive committee (MEC), as authorized by the hospital bylaws or other official documents (e.g., rules and procedures, standard operating procedures).[3]

Most institutions reserve a precautionary suspension as a last resort and typically prefer to go from informal warning (casually called "a coffee"), to a formal warning, typically in a written form, and then to a precautionary suspension.

The NPDB was created for a very specific reason: to protect patients from unsafe practice or practitioners. During a dispute, however, the NPDB can be used unfairly. The threat of a disciplinary action that will trigger an NPDB report is a major burden against a physician, but it is illegal to file a NPDB report for discriminatory or retaliatory reasons.

---

2 Berlin J. Under Investigation? Tex Med. 2017 Mar 01;113(3):49-53.

3 Snelson EA. National Practitioner Data Bank: more guidelines, more problems. Med Staff Couns. 1993 Summer;7(3):1-9. Pubmed

> **Health Care Quality Improvement Act of 1986** - Title I: Promotion of Professional Review Activities - Provides protection from liability under Federal and State laws for members of a professional review body and their staffs who, in the reasonable belief that the action was in the furtherance of quality health care, warranted by the facts known, and after a reasonable effort to obtain the facts, take actions which adversely affect the clinical privileges or professional society membership of a physician. Provides such protection to those who provide information to professional review bodies.[4]

In the US, the Health Care Quality Improvement Act (HCQIA) regulates the process of suspending or revoking one's clinical privileges. However, the institution involved is obligated to

- *notify you of any potential discipline and give you a right to a hearing before imposing such discipline*
- *make a "reasonable effort" to get the facts*
- *make a reasonable connection between those facts and the discipline it imposes.*

In most cases the hospital will attempt to connect the "offending behavior" to a safety risk; this is simply an attempt to follow a joint commission recommendation.[5]

---

4 [Health Care Quality Improvement Act of 1986]

5 (July 9, 2008: The Joint Commission Issued Sentinel Event Alert "Behaviors that Undermine a Culture of Safety").

Many institutions begin with a behind-the-scenes investigation and notifying the practitioner of a disciplinary action only after they've reached a preliminary decision. As a result, the hearing that follows is basically an appeal and the first chance to defend yourself.

At such a point, you shouldn't attempt to defend yourself without a lawyer. Investing into a good lawyer can make the difference between a clear record or an everlasting black dot on your profession and reputation with disastrous consequences for your future career, on that some lawyers like to call "irreparable injury."

Indeed, most institutions check the NPDB before making hiring decisions. Suspensions are also reported to your state licensing board. Moreover, the licensing board of every state has access to the NPDB. In some cases, the U.S. Drug Enforcement Agency and other bodies may also be alerted.

Let's be clear: some doctors whose privileges are revoked or suspended engage in truly improper behavior, such as:

- *interfering in a medical procedure and taking retaliatory steps to delay the delivery of healthcare;*[6]
- *providing substandard surgical care and falsifying medical records;*[7]
- *failing to order imaging before starting exploratory surgery and placing a catheter in an artery rather than a vein;*[8]
- *performing procedures that resulted in multiple patient deaths and injury, $1 million in malpractice liability and an adverse action by licensing authorities finding the doctor had acted with gross negligence;*[9]

---

6 Mahmoodian v United Hosp. Ctr., Inc., 185 W Va 59, 69, 404 SE2d 750, 760 [1991].

7 Hurwitz v AHS Hosp. Corp., 438 NJ Super 269, 284, 103 A3d 285, 294 [NJ Super Ct App Div 2014].

8 Urdinaran v Aarons, 115 F Supp 2d 484, 486 [DNJ 2000].

9 Chapman v Lourdes Med. Ctr. of Burlington County, A-0120-12T1, 2014 WL 4428248, at *1 [NJ Super Ct App Div Sept. 10, 2014].

- *deciding a patient needed surgery and then cancelling surgery without scheduling any further treatment when realizing the patient was not insured and the patient subsequently died;*[10]
- *harassing a patient by calling her on a weekend and aggressively criticizing another physician who was going to operate on her.*[11]

When You Take Legal Action

In case of a minor violation, you should discuss with your lawyer the possibility of a non-reportable suspension (less than 30 days), or suggest to get some extra education that would reassure your institution, such as a destressed or communication course with the aim to improve the physician' skills to deal with conflicts at work.

In case the due process requirements of the HCQIA were not followed, the action is unjustified, or the hospital's real motive is either discriminatory (racially targeting a doctor, for instance) or retaliatory (a reaction to your practice competing with another specialty, such as surgery, for instance), you have a real case for litigation if you cannot settle at the hospital level—whether a suspension by the hospital was enforced or not.

---

10 Ramamurthy v JFK Med. Ctr., A-4579-08T1, 2010 WL 2010993, at *4 [NJ Super Ct App Div May 21, 2010] (for this gross misconduct the surgeon received only a 90-day suspension of privileges).

11 Gordon v Lewistown Hosp., 423 F3d 184, 196 [3d Cir 2005].

Legal Cases When the Hospital Is Liable for False NPDN Reports

"Hospitals that create untrue NPDB reports may be liable for damages to the physicians reported. Although the Healthcare Quality Improvement Act may immunize hospitals and professional peer review bodies, those protections do not extend to peer reviews taken in bad faith or that do not comport with due process.

"In the case Sheikh v. Grant Regional Health Center (11-cv-1-wmc, W.D. Wisconsin), a Federal District Court denied a hospital's motion to dismiss claims for intentional infliction of emotional distress and negligent infliction of emotional distress, stating that a jury could infer that submitting false information to the National Practitioner Databank was intended to cause a physician severe emotional harm."[12]

- The court noted: "Knowingly publishing false information in a national database for the sole purpose of harming that person is the type of conduct that a reasonable jury could find to be extreme and outrageous."
- In addition: "A reasonable jury could certainly find a person has suffered 'an extreme disabling response' as a result of having false and disparaging information published about them on a national database and being precluded by that information from obtaining future employment in their chosen profession, par-

12 case Sheikh v. Grant Regional Health Center (11-cv-1-wmc, W.D. Wisconsin)

> ticularly if years were spent in qualifying one's self for that work."
>
> "Because damages in cases such as this may include a physician's past and future lost wages, the potential liability can be significant if a hospital loses such a case.
>
> "If a hospital threatens to report untrue or inaccurate information about a physician to the NPDB, the physician may help to establish a hospital's liability for doing so by putting the hospital on notice that the information is demonstrably false. Sending the hospital a certified letter or fax specifically stating how the proposed information is false and demanding that the hospital refrain from reporting the untrue information may be a deterrent to a hospital's bad behavior."[13]

In an ideal situation, where your case is straightforward, after being provided the claim(s), your lawyer can demonstrate during a fair hearing that your actions do not support suspension or, at worst, settle for a suspension that doesn't require NPDB reporting, hence less than 30 days. ***Remember that any settlement should include a retroactive change to your discipline below the NPDB's reporting threshold, so the hospital can void its report.***

In some cases, your lawyer might start litigating your discrimination or retaliation claim even as you cooperate in a fair hearing which threatens your clinical privileges. Indeed, ***filing a complaint at that***

---

13 https://sullivanlegal.us/hospital-may-be-liable-for-untrue-npdb-report/14 https://www.employmentlawgroup.com/in-the-news/articles/how-to-avoid-or-dispute-an-unfair-npdb-report/

point could give you leverage and allow you to request an injunction and maybe stop the current hearing altogether, without NPDB reporting.

If the institution is adamant about disciplinary action or your suspension has already started, your lawyer has 30 days to convince a judge that you have a valid claim, the hospital denied you certain rights and/or skipped certain steps according to their by-laws. You might prevail and have a judge issuing an order to stop the hospital from suspending your privileges and/or reporting action to the NPDB until you finish litigating your case, unless the hospital is able to demonstrate that there is an imminent risk to patients or staff.[14]

A Quick, Favorable Settlement?

Technically speaking, the moment a suspension is imposed, the physician's attorney will need to accomplish a huge amount of work in a very short time.[14] *This likely will include:*

- *An emergency motion for a temporary restraining order (TRO) and preliminary injunction (PI), to prevent defendant(s) from filing a report with the NPDB and to prevent defendant(s) from further disparaging the physician.*
    - *This emergency motion may also include a request to show cause why the TRO/PI should not be granted.*
- *Verified complaint*
- *Affidavits – physician's attorney, physician, and possibly experts and others*
- *Brief in support of the emergency motion.*

---

14 *Journal of American Physicians and Surgeons Volume 26 Number 3 Fall 2021*

The physician's attorney may also consider filing a Motion for Expedited Discovery, which in federal court is covered in Federal Rules of Civil Procedure (FRCP) Rule 26(d).[15] *The physician's attorney may obtain expedited discovery from the hospital to support his emergency motion for TRO/PI.*

The physician's attorney has subpoena power and can compel those who participated in the suspension at the hospital to testify at evidentiary hearings. This presents a valuable opportunity for the physician's attorney to lock down key testimony at an early stage, before these witnesses have had extensive coaching by the attorney representing the hospital.

The emergency motion for a TRO/PI will be followed by evidentiary hearings where each party argue why the TRO/PI should or should not be granted. These evidentiary hearings present the physician's attorney with an opportunity to put on his best case.

As one of the factors, the physician's attorney must prove to obtain a PI is a likelihood of prevailing on the merits, these evidentiary hearings can be seen as a mini-bench trial, a preview of the actual trial later. If the physician's attorney puts on a strong case, demonstrating likelihood that the physician will prevail on the case's merits, ***it is possible to achieve a favorable settlement at this stage. This saves the physician years of stress and tens of thousands (if not hundreds of thousands) of dollars.***

15 Majestro A. Preparing for and obtaining preliminary injunctive relief. Practice Points. American Bar Association; Jun 4, 2018. Available at: https://www.americanbar.org/groups/litigation/committees/woman-advocate/practice/2018/preliminary-injuction-relief/. Accessed Aug 12, 2021.

This pathway described above is unfortunately not known by most lawyers, which highlights the importance of selecting your lawyer very carefully. A defamation or employment lawyer might not be aware of this TRO/PI unique opportunity.

Such was the case of Dr. Fuentes's attorney, who let the 30 days deadline pass while waiting the end of a delayed investigation by the hospital to be completed.

After 30 Days

Once the action has been reported to the NPDB, typically after 30 days, things become more complicated. Regardless of what the institution has filed against you, you are allowed to add a supplemental statement online allowing anyone seeing your record to also see your version of the story. Nevertheless, your best option once reported is to obtain a complete removal or a "void" of the action. Unfortunately, this can only be performed by the institution which filed the report. Which means that you need to go through their lengthy process, which includes a hearing followed by an appeal first at the level of the MEC, then at the level of the Hospital board. Only after having exhausted all remedies internally are you then allowed to take your cases to court.

In the meantime, you can use the full extent of the law to protect your legal rights, for instance by suing a staff member for defamation (if a false claim was filed).

Another possibility is filing an official dispute, if the report was not submitted in accordance with NPDB's reporting regulations or didn't accurately depict the written report, or if the basis for the adverse action was not reflected in the written record provided by the reporting entity. Basically, a dispute addresses if the institution has filed their paperwork incorrectly.

Once a dispute has been filed, for a 60-day period, you should work with your institution to fix the problem. After that period ends, you must formally request escalation at the NPDB to request a correction.

If the dispute process doesn't end on your behalf, you could still proceed in federal court under the Administrative Procedures Act, but your chances of winning are limited.

Summary of the Administrative Procedure Act. 5 USC §551 et seq. (1946)

The Administrative Procedure Act (APA) governs the process by which federal agencies develop and issue regulations. It includes requirements for publishing notices of proposed and final rulemaking in the Federal Register, and provides opportunities for the public to comment on notices of proposed rulemaking. The APA requires most rules to have a 30-day delayed effective date.

In addition to setting forth rulemaking procedures, the APA addresses other agency actions such as issuance of policy statements, licenses, and permits. It also provides standards for judicial review if a person has been adversely affected or aggrieved by an agency action.

During the same time, your lawyer should still work to get your hospital to withdraw entirely your NPDB report. Once withdrawn, the NPDB will notify all state licensing bodies and tell agencies who queried your report to destroy any copies.

Unfortunately, even if you have a strong claim, your institution – for political or financial reasons, or in an attempt to eliminate competition – may not be interested about negotiating until the evening of a trial, so hire a strong lawyer and be prepared for a long and expensive fight.

The Suspension: Top 5 Takeaways

1. Your hospital can suspend you at any point, without previous notice, if they claim imminent danger to the health and/or safety of any individual or the organization.
2. Any suspension beyond 30 days is reportable to the NPDB
3. Only the institution can void a report filed in the NPDB
4. A NPDB report has disastrous consequences for the practitioner and can affect his professional career going forward overnight.
5. Hire a lawyer as soon as possible to work against the 30-day deadline.

CHAPTER 2

TWO MONTHS EARLIER: THE PERFECT STORM

To understand the situation of Dr. Fuentes, one needs to go back two months prior to the suspension, to a workday that culminated in "a perfect storm" of incidents that became the root of the precautionary suspension and all subsequent events.

The nursing director of the cath lab (Robert Blevins, RN) had taken a two-week vacation, leaving the unit in the hands of an interim manager (Christopher Simonar, RN). It is noteworthy to know that several physicians had already complained in the past to Robert about Christopher and his inability to manage the unit. Indeed, Christopher had few organizational skills and was unable to juggle the expectations of the nursing and physician staff.

That day, the cath lab was filled with patients scheduled for elective procedures to be dispatched between four rooms. Interventional rooms receive complex procedures such as coronarographies, percutaneous valves or pacemaker placements, among other procedures.

This particular morning was complicated by a cardiorespiratory arrest (or code) in a patient undergoing a coronarography, which required a team of providers form the intensive care unit (code team) to rush to the cath lab and begin immediate resuscitative efforts.

The patient was revived quickly and was waiting for a bed, nevertheless, nurse Christopher decided to send all nurses for a break, shutting down the unit for hours.

The remaining nurses were seen sitting around waiting for further instructions, some of them on their personal smartphones, texting or shopping online.

A lot of misconceptions exist related to a code situation. Once the code team has been called:

1. *Regular operation of the unit should resume if enough staff is available for the other rooms.*
2. *A code cart should allow for at least two codes to be managed at the same time, hence there is no need to wait to have several code carts on the unit.*

A modern cath lab requires the interaction of several services such as cardiology, anesthesia, nurse staff, housekeeping, and transportation.

In order to start a case in a typical cardiology suite, enough nurses and anesthesia support are required. By sending all nurses to a break, nurse Christopher Simonar made anesthesia support irrelevant, since nursing staff was no longer available. While Dr. Fuentes and his colleague, Dr. Anabella Strong, were able to secure enough support from anesthesia to resume procedures, no nursing staff was available.

Dr. Fuentes attempted to understand from nurse Christopher why he sent all the nursing staff to lunch without discussing with the cardiology leadership. He declined to provide a response and told him to contact her superior, the vice president of operations, Lara Malcom.

Dr. Fuentes left the unit and called VP Malcom to request her assistance in this matter. Dr. Fuentes came to learn from VP Malcom that Christopher had already taken a job as a nursing home nurse in the suburb of Phoenix and would be leaving the hospital by the end of the month.

In the meantime, Dr. Fuentes's partner, Dr. Strong, particularly upset about the total freeze of operations, decided to record a short videoclip of the staff sitting around shopping online. This started a cascade of events that would have a dramatic impact in the future.

The nurses noticed Dr. Strong recording a videoclip and immediately called security. Indeed, many hospitals have very strict guidelines about video recording, such that all people in the video need to consent for it and no patient or patient information can ever be on the clip. Security service came and obligated Dr. Strong to delete the video from her phone and verify that the video was also deleted from the deleted folder.

This sideshow event delayed operations in the cath lab even further. When Dr. Fuentes returned to the unit in the afternoon, the delay was so pronounced that several patients scheduled for elective procedures canceled or rescheduled. Around 4:00 PM, Dr. Fuentes wanted to see what inpatient he could bring down since the unit would be closing two rooms past 5:00 PM. He went to the unit desk to discuss with the afternoon charge nurse, Jane Clark. Dr. Fuentes was told that nurse Clark had called an intubated patient from the renal unit.

Dr. Fuentes was surprised to hear that Jane decided to call an intubated patient without checking with any of the physicians the priority order. In fact, due to the limited time remaining before rooms start closing, Dr. Fuentes wanted to postpone the intubated patient, who didn't require an emergent procedure, and proceed to a more urgent case. He attempted to understand why nurse Clark called the intubated patient, but Jane felt pressured and intimidated and started speaking over Dr. Fuentes to justify her mistake.

Seeing the escalation in her tone, Dr. Fuentes left the desk and called back VP Lara Malcom. He made sure the intubated patient was cancelled by his physician assistant Carmel Asuncion.

In the meantime, the interim manager, Christopher Simonar, went to the desk to discuss with Jane and decided to call security (again) as well as HR. Security services came briefly and left almost immediately without interrogating or discussing with any of the party, since there was no ongoing interaction between Dr. Fuentes and nurse Clark. The personal director, Clara Harari was the one who got the call from Christopher and went to speak to nurse Jane outside the unit. Jane was very agitated and could be heard across the wall, yelling that she is trying her best and nobody communicated with her, when in fact she was the one who failed to communicate to the different available physicians who to bring next to the unit.

Nurse Clark repeatedly said that she checked with Dr. Strong prior to calling the intubated patient, but Dr. Strong disagreed and confirmed Dr. Fuentes's claim that nurse Clark failed to communicate appropriately and tried to bring an intubated patient on her own initiative.

The next day an investigation was started by HR and interviewed the nurses involved in the morning event with the video taken by Dr. Strong and the four nurses present during the disagreement at the desk with nurse Clark.

Around the same time, Dr. Robert Grant, the chief of cardiology, the direct supervisor or Dr. Fuentes, was asked to do his own investigation by the medical leadership.

The Perfect Storm: Top 5 Takeaways

1. A perfect storm includes a combination of stressful situations and intense human interactions happening simultaneously.
2. Be aware of any strong reaction you might have and how it could be perceived.
3. Read the room in advance and keep your calm no matter what. Your ability of mastering your emotions will be instrumental for your future.
4. Avoid confrontation at all costs, especially during a patient safety matter.
5. Delegate rule enforcement or further actions to the respective supervisor or administrator.

CHAPTER 3

THE CONSPIRACY

HR's initial investigation stalled quickly, as soon as nurse Clark admitted twice in her deposition that Dr. Fuentes didn't yell at her but raised his voice and was condescending, while nurse Simonar filed a workplace violence complaint for the same incident. The rest of the nurses present during the interaction were not interested to expand on this non-significant event at that point.

In parallel, Dr. Grant finished his own investigation and summarized his findings in a statement provided to the Medical Executive Committee a couple days after the initial suspension of Dr. Fuentes. In his report he confirmed:

1. The lack of ability for the cath lab to deal appropriately with an emergency and running in an optimal fashion.
2. The poor turnover of the rooms in the cath lab, obligating the interventional team to stay late, to offer conflicting information to patients, and to cancel cases at the end of the day.
3. That the nurses didn't feel respected by the interventional team but confirmed that Dr. Fuentes didn't yell or threaten them but rather felt his manner was condescending or intimidating.

4. The unjustified filling of false claims of workplace violence by the nurses to destroy the physicians' reputation.

Things got quieter and seemed to be back to normal until the next Friday, when Nurse Simonar decided to shut down the unit for another three hours to celebrate a nurse's promotion. This time Dr. Fuentes decided to stay away from the unit while documenting to his superiors by email this retaliatory behavior.

The next week, Robert Blevins, the nurse director of the unit, was back from vacation and met with Dr. Fuentes, who told him that he was very disappointed in nurse Simonar's behavior and wanted to make sure he was never in charge of the cath lab until he left for his new job in the nursing home. He also shared with him the result of the turnover project and told him about his intention to present the data to the hospital leadership. Nurse Blevins was not happy about that idea since it could potentially demonstrate his poor leadership as a nursing director.

What Dr. Fuentes failed to recognize was that the two nurses (Blevins and Simonar) were very close and had already decided to use the system against him. Indeed, as soon as nurse Robert Blevins was back, he and nurse Simonar started solicitating nurses willing to speak to HR against Dr. Fuentes. Secret meetings were set up in the hospital library to recruit those nurses. A dozen nurses went, anonymously, to HR, including Robert and the VP Lara Malcolm, who felt the need to join this movement to secure her own job.

HR's initial, stalled investigation was suddenly refueled by a dozen nurses who narrated several undocumented disruptive events using key words to create a narrative compatible with breach of the "code of conduct." (see below).

Example Hospital Code of Conduct:

1. *Do not use offensive language, scream, or yell.*
2. *Do not use intimidation, foul language, or threats of violence or retaliation.*
3. *Do not discriminate on the basis of sex, religion, race, disability, age or sexual orientation.*
4. *Do not throw objects, engage in inappropriate touching, fighting or assault.*
5. *Do not harass others physically, verbally, psychologically, or sexually.*
6. *Do not retaliate against any individual who engages in activity protected under any federal, state, or local law.*
7. *Do not alter official documents and jeopardize the quality of care.*
8. *Do not mishandle, destroy, or steal hospital equipment.*
9. *Do not disregard safety rules and/or create a hazard.*
10. *Do not use or bring firearms, explosives, or any weapons on hospital property.*
11. *Do not refuse to obey Policies and Procedures.*
12. *Do not refuse to work cooperatively with other members of the Hospital.*

> *The creation of the code of conduct and its integration in the hospital bylaws is simply a reflection of the necessity for all major institutions to define unacceptable conduct.*

Nurse Robert Blevins then met with the VP of operations and claimed he wanted to resign due to the toxic and unsafe environment created by Dr. Fuentes. An emergency meeting was then called with the chairman of medicine, Dr. Friedland, who offered to set up a mediation meeting with Dr. Fuentes and Robert to resolve all issues.

But Robert preferred to meet with HR and was advised to file a corporate complaint—which he filed the day of Dr. Fuentes's suspension. It stated that Dr. Fuentes was taking video covering patient areas and creating a toxic working environment that was unsafe for staffs and patients.

> *A corporate complaint is the most serious complaint an employee can file, especially if the words "toxic environment" or "patient safety" are used in the claim.*

This complaint immediately triggered legal representation from the hospital against Dr. Fuentes. After the corporate complaint, the personnel director, Mrs. Clara Harari, was then able to request the precautionary suspension from the CMO and the medical staff president on the same day.

Over the course of the following week, several anonymous phone calls were made to the hospital hotline to report Dr. Fuentes—all after his suspension was made public. HR, under the direction of Mrs. Clara Harari, made sure to gather as many claims as it could to make sure Dr. Fuentes wouldn't come back

Understanding Legal Action: The Cat's Paw Theory

This conspiracy scenario is reminiscent of the cat's paw legal theory, in which an employer gets the legal blame even if the actual executive or supervisor who fires or demotes a physician does not act out of a biased intent but rather the bias of another executive or supervisor who informed the final decision (in this case the nurse leadership of the cath lab).[16]

The "cat's paw" theory gets its name from a fable, written in 1679 by the French poet Jean de La Fontaine, about a monkey who persuaded a cat to pull chestnuts out of a fire—the cat gets burned and the monkey makes off with the chestnuts.

The "cat's paw" theory of liability falls upon the employer only if these steps play out in a sequence:

1. *a person in a leadership position takes a step – in this case the personnel director, the medical staff president and/or the chief medical office along with the MEC (starting a suspension process) – that is done for a biased reason;* ***which in this case is the one created by a conspiracy from a group of nurses, a nurse director, a manager, and a VP of operations.***
2. *the leadership representative intends to get the physician fired, demoted, or otherwise penalized, and*
3. *the leader's step is found to be the "proximate" cause of the ultimate decision — even if the executive or supervisor who actually carries out the firing or other penalty is someone else, and that person was not at all biased.*

---

16 *Pipal, Bill; Robbennolt, Jennifer K. (2011). "Court rules on 'cat's paw' theory of discrimination". Monitor on Psychology. Retrieved 2023-03-25.*

Hence, even if the medical executive committee were to do an investigation before acting, it would not neutralize the effect of the other supervisors' bias and doesn't get the hospital off the hook based on the precedent of federal cases.[17,18]

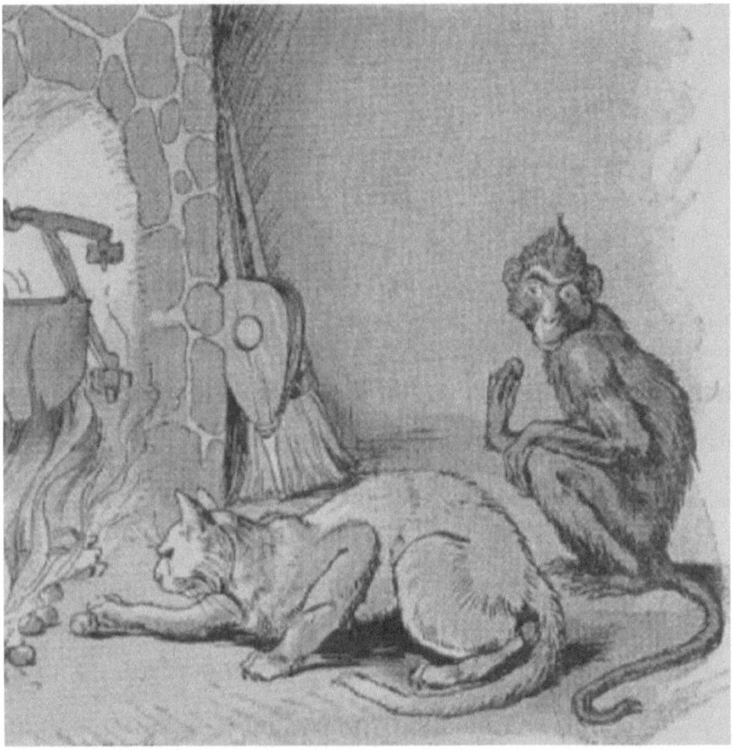

17 *See e.g.,* Meade v Twp. of Livingston, 249 NJ 310, 336, 265 A3d 148, 163-64 [2021] ("Unlawful employment discrimination -- whether based on gender or on the exercise of protected conduct -- can be predicated on claims that a non-decision maker's discriminatory views impermissibly influenced the decision maker to take an adverse employment action against an employee. In other words, actions taken to accommodate discriminatory views can support liability to the same extent as actions taken based on personally held discriminatory views.");

18 Staub v Proctor Hosp., 562 US 411, 421, 131 S Ct 1186, 1193, 179 L Ed 2d 144 [2011]("But if the independent investigation relies on facts provided by the biased supervisor—as is necessary in any case of cat's-paw liability—then the employer (either directly or through the ultimate decision maker) will have effectively delegated the fact finding portion of the investigation to the biased supervisor.").

The Conspiracy: Top 5 Takeaways

1. Be aware of your institution's code of conduct.
2. Claims are nowadays captured in a computerized manner by human resources.
3. Every claim ever filed against you, investigated or not, is retrievable by your administration at any time.
4. Workplace violence is a serious claim that can be made against you without any proof of veracity required.
5. The institution is liable for its legal action against you even if it was lured into the action by some of its personnel.

CHAPTER 4

ONE WEEK POST-SUSPENSION: THE MEDICAL EXECUTIVE COMMITTEE HEARING

The day after his suspension, Dr. Fuentes requested via email a meeting to meet with the members of the medical executive committee (MEC). He then received electronically a letter confirming a meeting with the MEC to discuss the circumstances surrounding his precautionary suspension. Interestingly, no details as to why Dr. Fuentes was suspended were provided in the letter.

Dr. Fuentes was allowed to bring an attorney, who could advise him but could not speak. So he went to the meeting with his lawyer, Alan Rogers, at the time provided in the letter.

The amphitheater was arranged for the MEC meeting. Tables were placed in a circle and took up the whole available space, leaving a vacuum in the center. There was close to thirty people seated, including the medical staff president, the CMO, and most medical chiefs (Internal Medicine, Surgery, Cardiothoracic Services, Gynecology, Oncology Services, Colo-rectal Services, and so on).

At his entrance into the auditorium, Dr. Fuentes was given a large file containing the issues to be presented. He then had a few minutes to review it before his appearance in front of the MEC. As he flipped through the file, which had redacted the names of those who provided testimony against him, it sunk in that the summary placed on top of the file was about him creating a toxic environment and breaching the code of conduct in correlation mainly with the "perfect storm" event and a history of "disruptive behavior."

The file also contained every single complaint filed against him over the years, most of them without his knowledge, and many in duplicate and even triplicate. What was very concerning to him was the fact that none of the complaint resolutions or his own responses to those known complaints were included. It became clear that this file was created to take him down.

He was invited to sit down with his lawyer and then watched to his surprise as the personnel director, Mrs. Clara Harari, entered the room and was asked to present the case against him by the medical staff president, Dr. Marie Rattner.

It is very unusual for Human Resources to give the leading presentation against a physician. Most MEC prefer a physician to perform this difficult task. Indeed, HR can be biased against physicians, especially if they represent mainly non-physician staff (nurses, technicians, etc.).

He listened to Mrs. Clara Harari's presentation and heard about a physician (him) yelling, screaming, and terrorizing his nurses and colleagues, and putting patients' lives in danger by doing dangerous procedures, **sometimes without their consents.**[19]

Dr. Fuentes was dizzy and nauseated to hear all those false accusations. At the end of this surreal presentation, he was asked to speak.

Dr. Fuentes took a deep breath and started by explaining exactly what happened on the day of the "perfect storm." He denied the yelling, screaming, and abusing of nurses. He insisted that he was not present during the video taking and all that happened was a disagreement in the afternoon at the desk of the cath lab. He clarified that there were never any safety issues, and totally objected to the statement of endangering patients or doing procedures without consent. He insisted that he always had an open-door policy and allowed cross check during any procedures by anyone in the cath lab, whether physicians, nurses, or technicians.

Dr. Fuentes went on to say that any time you create a new program, you need to go through the motions of educating the staff and making sure other disciplines slowly accept your program and vision. He reminded everyone that he spearheaded several meetings and created several algorithms allowing relations with other disciplines (such as cardiothoracic surgery and anesthesia) to dramatically improve over the years.

At the end of his presentation, several members started asking him questions. He was asked up front if he was *remorseful*, which

---

19 Doing procedure without consent can be considered battery. Ref: https://notputtingonashirt.org/2018/09/18/informed-consent-the-difference-between-medical-care-and-battery/

basically implied that he was guilty. He was asked why he recorded that video (even though he wasn't the one who recorded the video) and why so many complaints were filed against him. He tried to explain that as a leader of the group, he represented his partner several times in difficult conversations with other services, in the best interest for the patients, while always following the code of conduct.

Despite his explanations, it became clear to Dr. Fuentes that the minds of those on the executive committee were set. The size of the file and the damming presentation by the personnel director, Mrs. Clara Harari, had already misled them and determined his fate.

He was asked to leave and was told that they will be calling him.

The rest of the meeting was behind closed doors. An insider later told Dr. Fuentes what transpired. What started as a complaint from a group of nurses suddenly became an opportunity for cardiothoracic surgery to finally get rid of Dr. Fuentes.

It is important to remember that since his arrival at the hospital, Dr. Fuentes and his team took over the care of many cardiac patients previously managed by cardiothoracic surgery by offering minimally invasive treatment. This had led to several conflicts between the two disciplines in the past and necessitated the introduction of a mediation process by the previous CMO, Dr. Rafael Navin, in which any party (interventional cardiology or cardiothoracic surgery) could call a mediator to facilitate resolution of a clinical issue in case of clinical disagreement.

The chair of surgery (Dr. Christina Taley) and medicine (Dr. Friedland) sparred about what to do with Dr. Fuentes. The chair of medicine defended Dr. Fuentes and insisted on the difficulties of changing a culture and starting a challenging program in a new environment. He conceded that Dr. Fuentes might be perceived difficult by some, but he was a passionate physician and dedicated leader.

The chair of surgery, backed by the nurse union representative (Nurse Olivia Grogun), insisted that Dr. Fuentes was incapable of interacting appropriately with other disciplines and seemed to be remorseless of his actions. They couldn't see him coming back to work just after a warning—something more drastic needed to be done, in the face of such grave accusations, she said as she pointed at the large file created by HR.

The MEC members voted unanimously to continue the suspension and create a special committee to investigate Dr. Fuentes.

Hindsight is 20/20

Looking back, Dr. Fuentes should have had a different attitude during the meeting with the MEC. He should have requested the MEC to spell out the exact reason of his suspension and what he was being accused off. There was no need for him to speak or explain anything if no explanation was provided to him prior.

At the same time, the file that was handed to him and the MEC was too large to be assessed thoroughly, hence he should have requested more time to assess and provide a rebuttal. This would have probably led to the same result in prolongation of the suspension, but at least he would avoid the perception of his attempt to defend himself as exhibiting a lack of remorse or awareness.

The MEC Committee Hearing: Top 5 Takeaways

1. The medical executive meeting can sustain or vacate a suspension.
2. Insist on knowing the exact accusations brought against you.
3. In front of the MEC or hospital board, the less you speak, the better.
4. Take note of the presentation given to the MEC, since you won't have access to any discovery later.
5. Bring your lawyer—even if he is not allowed to speak to the MEC members, he can still advise you.

CHAPTER 5

WHAT TO DO DURING A HOSPITAL INVESTIGATION

Once suspended, most institutions will start a peer-related investigation if the allegations are not clear or require more tangible proofs. ***Please be aware that a major violation of the bylaws or the code of conduct might result in an immediate revocation of privileges or termination.*** *For example: video footage of a physician physically pushing another physician or staff during a procedure, (even if it's meant to be related to training, supervision, or proctoring) or any act of violence captured on camera.*

An investigation at the hospital level can take up to 90 days. The first two months of suspension are probably the hardest ones. Indeed, in most cases, the physician is totally kept in the dark while awaiting the result of the investigation. Many institutions, under the pretext of protecting some individuals from retaliation, would not disclose any information related to the individual or individuals who put forward the original claim. This makes the task of the physician trying to defend himself extremely difficult.

The institution also will typically remove your access to the electronic medical record, making it impossible for you to interact with your patients anymore.

Some key advice you need to follow in order to get through this difficult phase:

1. ***Hire an experienced lawyer, ideally a healthcare lawyer.*** *This seems pretty straight forward, especially if the suspension is going to last 30 days or more (hence become reportable to the NPDB). You might be tempted to resolve this suspension quickly and show how compliant you are in order to come back to work quickly, however be very careful what you say or what you write from this point on.* ***Indeed, any admission of guilt or remorse can be used against you in the future. Some friends or colleagues might advise (unwisely) you to call, write, or email to apologize, but don't even think about it without legal advice.*** *Don't settle quickly in order to avoid expensive legal bills—this is your career, your name, and your reputation being threatened, and those are priceless.*
2. ***Under no circumstances should you resign.*** *Doing so will have a disastrous impact on your career and future as a clinician. The NPDB is very clear about that concept:* ***"a surrender of clinical privileges or failure to renew clinical privileges while under investigation or to avoid investigation must be reported."***
3. ***Try to keep your license(s) current and valid,*** *in order to be able to secure another job if needed. Remember, most licensing boards are mainly concerned about a violation at work if is related to a sexual offense, patient safety, or a performance issue.*
4. ***Try to keep access, if possible, to your work email.*** *Indeed, doing so will allow you not only to be informed about daily activities of the institution suspending you but will also provide you with invaluable access to sign-outs, previously sent emails to key individuals, and communications about the potential transfers, resig-*

nations, and other events related directly or indirectly to your case.

5. *From this point on,* ***be very careful about your phone calls and text messaging to any people at work****. These might be retrievable if you go to a civil and/or federal court.*
6. *If you know or suspect the nature of the claims made against you,* ***start immediately doing your homework****. For instance:*
   - *Find out if a video was taken of the event; this can literally save your case and totally exonerate you.* ***An orthopedic surgeon was accused by a nurse of pushing her on the stairs and was subsequently arrested and taken to jail by the local police. A camera in the stairs demonstrated that the nurse lied and she ended up being fired while the physician was reinstated with apology from the hospital.***[20]
   - *Retrieve emails related to the incident and save them as a PDF with dates and details of whom it was sent to.*
   - *Extract texts capturing your communications related to your case and save them as well as PDFs.*
   - *Seek written testimonies from people witness to those events or incidents. You can also contact people who can speak to your character in writing. You won't be able to seek those testimonies from people still working at the hospital, but you should be able to request them from those who previously worked with you. You can either have those statements notarized or add this specific sentence at the end of their letter.*

     "I declare under penalty of perjury that the foregoing is true and correct.
     Executed on (date)
     (Signature)"

---

20 A similar case, settled outside of court, with no further references available: https://www.seattletimes.com/nation-world/charges-dropped-against-surgeon-accused-of-assaulting-nurse/#:~:text=Charges%20dropped%20against%20surgeon%20accused%20of%20assaulting%20nurse%20%7C%20The%20Seattle%20Times

7. ***Take care of yourself.*** *Eat healthy, work out, find support with your significant other and/or your friends, take some time off, and spend quality time with your family. Most institutions would not suspend your salary, at least not immediately, so this should allow you to take some well-deserved time off.*
8. ***Seek therapy.*** *Don't let depression, anxiety, fear, and lack of sleep take the best of you. Suicide has been described (see references) in physicians in such proceedings, so do not let yourself become a victim of a flawed system.*[21,22,23,24,25,26,27,28,29,30]
9. ***Maintain your clinical privileges*** *by doing all the required HIPAA training; flu and Covid vaccinations, etc. Don't give your institution any excuses to get rid of you for not following their mandated regulations or trainings.*

---

21 Spiers C. Suicide in the workplace. Occup Health. (Lond). 1996;48(7):247-249.

22 Kaufmann M. Physician suicide: risk factors and prevention. Ont Med Rev. 2000, 67(8):20–22.

23 Schernhammer ES, Colditz GA. Suicide rates among physicians: a quantitative and gender assessment (meta-analysis). Am J Psychiatry. 2004;161:295–302.

24 4 Worley L, Our fallen peers: a mandate for change. Acad Psychiatry. 2008;32:1,8-12.

25 Hampton T. Experts address risk of physician suicide. JAMA. 2005;294:1189–1191.

26 Hendin H, Reynolds C, Fox D., et.al. Licensing and physician mental health: problems and possibilities. J Medical Licensure & Discipline. 2007;93:8-11.

27 Noovsa, D. Doctors Who Kill Themselves. [Newsweek Web site]. April 28, 2008;151(17):16. Available at: http://www.newsweek.com/id/132887. Accessed June 18, 2008.

28 Noonan, D. Doctors Who Kill Themselves. [Newsweek Web site]. April 28, 2008;151(17):16. Available at: http://www.newsweek.com/id/132887. Accessed June 18, 2008.

29 Givens J, Tjia J. Depressed medical students' use of mental health services and barriers to use. Acad Medicine. 2002;77:918-921

30 Crawford, NS. The road to recovery: training to help the impaired pharmacist. Am Pharm. 1991;NS31(5):33-5, 38.

10. ***Keep practicing your craft,*** *especially if you are a procedural physician or need financial compensation for your legal fees. But more importantly, it is crucial that you maintain your skills. This can be realized in several different manners.*
    - *Volunteer in foreign countries. Indeed, some countries are in need of people with your skills and volunteering would dramatically benefit the local population.*
    - *Publish those papers that have been sitting on your desktop for lack of time.*
    - *Explore the options of locum tenens or per diem, although some locum tenens might not hire you once the NPDB filling has been provided to them. But this doesn't discourage you to try—some remote places are in need of physicians and willing to hire you as long as you can convince them that you don't pose a threat to their patients and staff.*
11. ***Discuss with a financial adviser,*** *the best option to pay your lawyer,* many physicians have live insurance with access to immediate cash value whenever an urgent financial need comes up, this is extremely useful since it avoids lapidation of one's retirement during this process. Another option would be to take a loan. It is crucial then to pay your monthly fees on time to prevent damaging your credit score.
12. Start mak*ing a list of how this suspension has created "irreparable damages."*
    - *Capture communications of patients contacting you for being unable to see you.*
    - *Sum-up all patient appointments canceled or rescheduled.*
    - *Add up total amount of money spent on legal fees and psychiatry.*
    - *Have your financial adviser estimate the real monetary damage in case you use your savings or live insurance cash value.*

- *List all opportunities declining to hire you due to the NPDB filing.*
- *Capture communications with state licensing authorities and insurance related to the suspension and NPDB filing.*
- *Have your psychiatrist describe the psychological harm done to you during this process.*
- *Document all false rumors spread regarding the cause of your suspension and their consequences (inability to find a job, being invited to a regional or national course, etc.)*

13. ***Don't blame yourself.*** *The hospital treating you this way is trying to convince you that you have done something wrong, so they can make you "bend the knee." Indeed, most hospital bylaws are designed to punish the physician by forcing them into a long and expensive process that leads them to either bankruptcy, if they want to exert their rights, or settling, by waving their hearing right, exposing them to all kinds of unjustified sanctions.*

    You must remember, again and again, that an institution that tolerates both false allegations and the individuals who feel safe to make them are the problem, not the doctor who fights back against defamatory charges.

14. *Be aware that* ***at some point the leadership that has hired you and supported you will abandon you****. Indeed, once they see that you intend to exert all your rights (to a hearing and appeal), you will become "radioactive." They will stop responding to your calls or emails and they will focus on preserving the service you created or developed. They will start reaching out to your partners and offer them salary raises and promotions to take over your patients and/or your titles.*
15. Expect the reactions of colleagues during this process to be classified into three different categories.

A. *Some will simply vaporize, scared by the different rumors spreading about your suspension and will want nothing to do with you during that process. Most people will fall in this category.*

B. *A few will support you and will become crucial during an appeal or a hearing procedure. The amount of people willing to support you during this process speaks to your character and will be instrumental during a hearing (see chapter 9).*

C. *A final few might turn against you and see this as an opportunity to finally give you "a coup de grace." These are typically competing physicians or physicians you have been in conflict with in the past, but also be ready to experience betrayal from people you called "professional friends." These are perhaps the worst people, who in exchange for a promotion or recognition would gladly testify against you.*

For those colleagues testifying against another physician, a few pieces of advice:

1. ***The hospital lawyers are not your lawyer, they will use you to achieve their aim (i.e., protect the hospital).***
2. ***Anything you might say can be retrieved and used against you in a defamation lawsuit, especially if your statement was the basis of a sanction against a practitioner.***
3. ***There is no obligation for you to testify at the hospital level unless you receive a subpoena.***
4. ***If you end up testifying against a colleague, be extremely careful what you say. Avoid at all costs making blunt and definitive statements and under no circumstances make it personal. This is not your career on the line but that of another practitioner who went through the same struggles as you did to become a licensed physician.***

The Special Committee's Investigation

After the special committee was created, its four members started reviewing all of the documents provided and decided who besides the defendant they intended to interview.

> *A fair process typically involves several people to be interviewed and review of all claims and videos potentially available.*

The investigators decided to extract all complaints filed against Dr. Fuentes and went as far back as six years. They were not provided, nor requested, the resolution(s) of each complaint. It is likely that the investigators obtained legal counsel in seeking to justify the suspension.

Problems started to arise when the four members were not available for all interviews, or when poor documentation of interviews were captured, especially if an interview was positive, while emphasis was put on negative interviews.

In one case, a very antagonistic physician to Dr. Fuentes was interviewed at the same time as a neutral one, which lead to interference in the testimonies captured. Indeed, the neutral practitioner became clearly influenced by the antagonist physician and didn't dare to say anything positive on Dr. Fuentes's behalf to avoid offending his colleague.

In addition, some positive interviews were not documented appropriately or were omitted altogether from the final report. Negative testimonies were given more importance in time and content and some statements were even reversed/altered to blame Dr. Fuentes. Indeed, a nurse who was specifically asked "did Dr. Fuentes create an 'us versus them culture,'" said "no;" but in the final conclusion of the report, it had her saying, "Dr. Fuentes created an 'us versus them' culture."

What to Do during a Hospital Investigation: Top 5 Takeaways

1. An investigation can take up to three months and most probably will be reported to the NPDB.
2. Any signs that the hospital lawyers are involved should raise a red flag.
3. Do your own homework, gather your own evidence.
4. As tempting as it seems, do not bend the knee or resign.
5. Take care of yourself.

CHAPTER 6

THE END OF PHYSICIAN LEADERSHIP AND THE CONCEPT OF "DISRUPTIVE BEHAVIOR"

It is important to remember one of the most important paradigm shifts since the beginning of the century: ***the end of physician leadership****.*

The oldest physicians currently practicing were trained or grew up in a time where leaders in healthcare were physicians, just like them. Physicians today have become so busy dealing with their patients, documentation, coding, and more that they have failed to pay attention to who has taken over their own control.

Increasingly over the past decade, physicians have given away their leadership position quietly without any complains or struggle.[31] *Some might call it a "silent takeover." Leadership in healthcare is now in*

31 **Sponsored by VMG Health | info@vmghealth.com | 214.369.4888 Physicians are losing power. Here's why. Patsy Newitt - Thursday, June 8th, 2023

the hand of financially-trained persons, unions, nurses with degrees in healthcare or economics, and lawyers with business degrees or backgrounds.[32]

At the same time, the number of administrators has risen at a much more rapid rate than the number of physicians, along with an increase in related rules, regulations, and management procedures.[33]

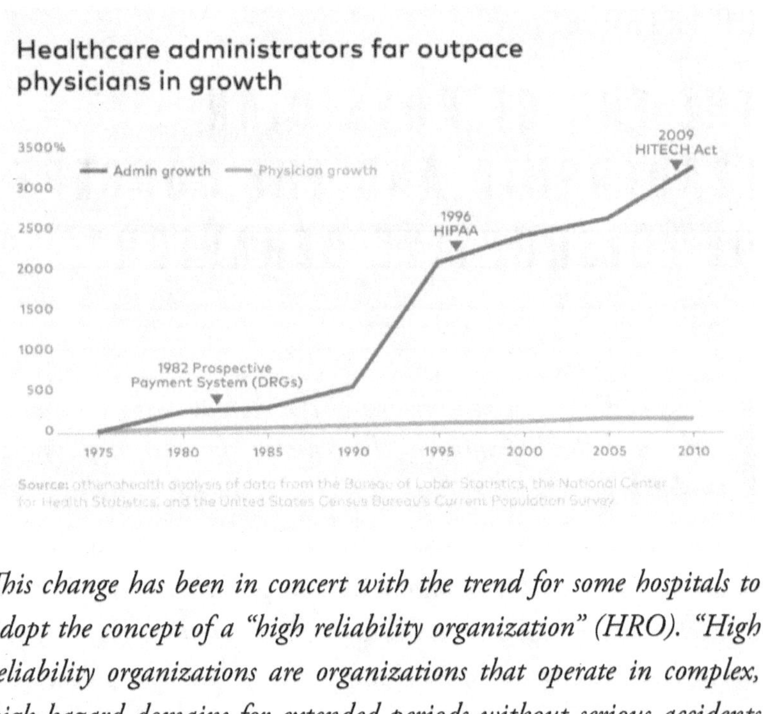

This change has been in concert with the trend for some hospitals to adopt the concept of a "high reliability organization" (HRO). "High reliability organizations are organizations that operate in complex, high-hazard domains for extended periods without serious accidents or catastrophic failures. The concept of high reliability is attractive for health care, due to the complexity of operations and the risk of sig-

---

32 ***https://well.blogs.nytimes.com/2011/07/07/should-hospitals-be-run-by-doctors/

33 https://www.athenahealth.com/knowledge-hub/practice-management/expert-forum-rise-and-rise-healthcare-administrator#:~:text=Here's%20some%20food%20for%20thought,for%20the%20same%20time%20period.

nificant and even potentially catastrophic consequences when failures occur in health care. Sometimes people interpret high reliability as meaning effective standardization of health care processes. However, the principles of high reliability go beyond standardization; high reliability is better described as a condition of persistent mindfulness within an organization. High reliability organizations cultivate resilience by relentlessly prioritizing safety over other performance pressures."[34]

At the same time, the corporatization of medicine has had a subsequent impact on physicians and their interactions with one another.[35] *Instead of collaborating, physicians are competing with each other.*

While the medical field has always been prone to competition—in medical school, residency, and fellowship, and at every stage of their career—physicians traditionally learned to compete to progress to the next step or to be promoted.

But the competition utilized by large corporations today incentivizes physicians based on their productivity, especially in the surgical or procedure-driven specialties. Plus, the development of minimally invasive procedures has de facto created opposing trends between several specialties of surgery and interventional cardiology, neurology gastroenterology, or pulmonary, which added to the competition among physicians.

To make things worse, physicians have never been prone to being unionized, which makes them extremely week to defend themselves against large corporations when compared to nurses' union, for instance.[36]

---

34 https://psnet.ahrq.gov/primer/high-reliability

35 https://www.nytimes.com/2023/05/21/opinion/letters/health-care-corporations.html

36 Three reasons why doctors don't unionize Baird Brightman, PHD Policy July 10, 2020

On Disruptive Behaviors

"In 2009, The Joint Commission (TJC) began to address 'disruptive behaviors.' Disruptive behavior includes aggressive behavior such as yelling, foul and abusive language, threatening gestures, public criticism of coworkers, insult and shaming, intimidation, invading one's space, slamming down objects, and other physically aggressive behavior. It also includes passive-aggressive behaviors such as hostile avoidance or the "cold shoulder" treatment, intentional miscommunication, unavailability for professional matters, e.g., not answering pages or delays in doing so, speaking in a low or muffled voice, condescending language or tone, impatience with questions, malicious gossip, racial, gender, sexual, or religious slurs or "jokes", jokes" about a person's personal appearance, sarcasm, implied threats, especially retribution for making complaints.[37]

The American Medical Association defined inappropriate behavior as conduct that is unwarranted and is reasonably interpreted to be demeaning or offensive. Persistent, repeated inappropriate behavior can become a form of harassment and thereby become disruptive, and subject to treatment as "disruptive behavior."

While disruptive behavior means any abusive conduct, including sexual or other forms of harassment, or other forms of verbal or non-verbal conduct that harms or intimidates others to the extent that quality of care or patient safety could be compromised. (The term of "disruptive physician" is a term often used in lectures, publications, or discussion, although some institutions prefer to stay away from it nowadays.)

---

37 *https://www.foley.com/en/insights/publications/2008/07/the-joint-commissions-sentinel-event-alert-on-disr*

See AMA Code of Medical Ethics §9.4.4: "The importance of respect among all health professionals as a means of ensuring good patient care is foundational to ethics. Physicians have a responsibility to address situations in which individual physicians behave disruptively, that is, speak or act in ways that may negatively affect patient care, including conduct that interferes with the individual's ability to work with other members of the health care team, or for others to work with the physician. Disruptive behavior is different from criticism offered in good faith with the aim of improving patient care and from collective action on the part of physicians. Physicians must not submit false or malicious reports of disruptive behavior."[38]

The two key concepts of disruptive behavior to remember: ***their repetitive pattern combined with the potential that the quality of care or patient/staff safety could be compromised.*** *In order for a healthcare institution to capture those patterns, documentation is essential.*

Electronic reporting has *bridged that gap by allowing anonymous and seamless reporting of those" alleged" behaviors. Some reporting platforms have a "workplace violence" section that could be filled online. The only caveat is the veracity of those complaints—anyone can file anything about anyone without any cross check (see chapter 2).*[39]

---

38 https://code-medical-ethics.ama-assn.org/sites/default/files/2022-08/9.4.4.pdf See *Disruptive Physician Behavior,* Journal of Medical Regulation, Vol. 98 No.1

39 Sham Peer Review: Abuse of Incident Reporting Software. Journal of American Physicians and Surgeons Volume 27 Number 3 Fall 2022

Disruptive Behavior?

In the case of Dr. Fuentes's "disruptive behavior," the following complaints were used by the hospital to suspend him. It's noteworthy that when the hospital discussed this case, it didn't include any discussion of the below resolutions to each complaint. Any negative interaction documented in the system was used against him, in particular:

- One professional disagreement with a general cardiologist who consulted cardiothoracic surgery on a patient of Dr. Fuentes without his knowledge. The patient was responding to minimally invasive cardiac therapy and was sent for an unnecessary operation. (This incident was resolved after discussion with the supervisor of the general cardiologist and was witnessed by the PA of Dr. Fuentes.)
- Several professional interactions concerning disagreements at the cath lab front desk between Dr. Fuentes and a charge nurse, each submitted in duplicate and inaccurately converted into incidents. (Multiple sworn testimonies provided by people working daily with Dr. Fuentes contradict the claims in these statements.)
- One interaction related to an incident with an anesthesiologist refusing to start a case and grabbing Dr. Fuentes's phone while he was discussing with his supervisor. (This was investigated in-depth by an independent investigator with exoneration of Dr. Fuentes and with the anesthesiologist found to be not credible.)
- One difficult interaction with cardiothoracic surgery, which was submitted in duplicate, related to a patient of Dr. Fuentes who was inappropriately sent to surgery and subsequently died. (This led to a meeting with the involved services as well

as hospital leadership with a resolution that future differences in opinion on patient management between the interventional cardiology group and cardiothoracic surgery should be resolved by a designated mediator with establishment of an algorithm of treatment and steps to be followed.)

- One interaction with a hospitalist, regarding a difference of opinion in the management of a patient of Dr. Fuentes's. (The hospitalist admitted later under oath to have lost his cool and yelled.)
- One interaction, submitted in duplicate, regarding an anesthesiologist wanting to place an arterial line inappropriately on a patient, putting the patient at unnecessary risk. (This is cleared in a document provided by the superior of the anesthesiologist and witnessed by a colleague of Dr. Fuentes.)
- One interaction with an anesthesiologist delaying a case and claiming Dr. Fuentes was invading her space while Dr. Fuentes was simply handing her his mobile to connect her with the surgeon on call, as requested by the anesthesiologist. (This was investigated in-depth with total exoneration of Dr. Fuentes and the anesthesiologist's claim found to be not credible.)
- One incident with cardiothoracic surgery.' This was related to a patient of Dr. Fuentes nearly being taken to surgery without discussion with Dr. Fuentes. (This patient ended up declining surgery and responding to minimally invasive treatment proposed by Dr. Fuentes. This incident was witnessed as a professional interaction by a colleague, a PA, and investigated with total exoneration of Dr. Fuentes.)
- One incident with cardiothoracic surgery. The surgery team did not communicate with Dr. Fuentes team about a shared patient prior to taking them to surgery, and filed a claim when Dr. Fuentes asked them to hold off on surgery until

he communicated with the designated mediator as per the agreed upon protocol for when there was a difference in opinion on patient management (see earlier).

- One incident, submitted by cardiothoracic surgery, about a shared patient who was taken to surgery in disregard of the protocol to communicate with the designated mediator when there was a difference in opinion on patient management. This was documented in an email by the mediator, supporting Dr. Fuentes to surgical and medical leadership.
- One phone conversation with a cardiothoracic surgeon during which Dr. Fuentes agreed for the patient to go for surgery but requested an intraoperative coronarogram during surgery. The conversation documented in the claim stating Dr. Fuentes refused the patient to go to surgery was inaccurate. (This conversation was witnessed by Dr. Fuentes's physician assistant.)
- Eight unrelated claims concerning: defective devices, a malfunctioning monitor, an outpatient clinic appointment delay, a patient being admitted to the wrong service, an unawareness of a patient admission, a delay in a patient's procedure due to lack of space, and difficulty in ordering a device. (None of those should have been included.)

A thorough examination of those claims demonstrates:

1. **Many claims were submitted twice, and some claims even submitted three times.**
2. **All included claims were resolved, investigated, unrelated, or irrelevant, and do not justify Dr. Fuentes's suspension.**
3. **There is no pattern of disruptive behavior but rather a toxic tendency to weaponize the reporting system.**

4. **There was no patient-safety concern in the included claims. On the contrary, Dr. Fuentes consistently advocated for his patients with the aim to prevent unnecessary procedures. Even when he followed the agreed-upon protocol to consult a mediator during differences of opinion on patient management with cardiothoracic surgery, he was still reported against.**
5. **No other surgeons whom Dr. Fuentes works with consistently had filed claims against him other than cardiothoracic surgery (e.g., surgical oncology, colorectal surgery, thoracic surgery, general surgery, pediatric surgery as well as urology). This suggests a communication concern with cardiothoracic** surgery rather than with Dr. Fuentes.

The End of Physician Leadership: Top 5 Takeaways

1. Physicians have lost leadership of the hospital, while the number of administrators has steadily risen.
2. Hospital leadership is in the hand of financial experts, lawyers, and/or hospital staff with business degrees.
3. Disruptive behaviors have received extreme scrutiny by the Joint Commission and the AMA.
4. Only the repetitive pattern and/or its association with patient and/or staff safety allow the hospital to act against the practitioner.
5. Electronic reporting allows seamless documentation of any behavior—*by* anyone and *about* anyone—without providing any proof of veracity.

CHAPTER 7

THE RECOMMENDATION OF THE MEDICAL EXECUTIVE COMMITTEE

After three months of investigations, the MEC received an investigation summary from the special committee. Twenty-four hours later, a presentation to the MEC was then given during an extraordinary session.

The investigation report was not provided to Dr. Fuentes immediately—it took three additional weeks before the report was released to him.

Dr. Fuentes expected to be reinstated. He knew that there was nothing that justified the suspension. Over the last three months, the two main accusers had already left the cath lab. Indeed, Nurse Simonar left to join a nursing home, while Nurse Robert Blevins was pushed to the geriatric clinics by hospital leadership, which led Dr. Fuentes to think that the investigation confirmed the conspiracy led by nurse Blevins and Simonar to get rid of him.

At the extraordinary session of the medical executive committee, the report was read out to the MEC, first covering all the parties interviewed. Paradoxically, the majority of the people interviewed supported Dr. Fuentes.

Nevertheless, the four-person investigative committee found enough proof to justify the initial suspension since failure to do so might, according to them, have posed a danger to any individual or the operation of the hospital. The investigative committee also felt that Dr. Fuentes's lacked insight about his behaviors--as he instead focused on the resolution of each incident than the trigger itself—basically placing the blame for every interaction on him.

Most concerning was the acknowledgment that even though several specialists (interventional radiologists, oncologists, general surgeons, and emergency physicians) were supportive, others specialties felt that interactions with Dr. Fuentes challenged their ability to care for patients and prevented them from requesting consultation with him. Nevertheless, everyone agreed that Dr. Fuentes's skillset is quite unique and beneficial to many patients.

For several members of the MEC, it was clear from its tone that the report was not presented in a balanced manner, but rather sought to portray Dr. Fuentes in the most unfavorable way possible and downplayed any information that was favorable to him. The "perfect storm" event was not even mentioned, and the focus had clearly shifted to past events—even though these had been investigated, resolved, or deemed irrelevant at the time.

Many members of the MEC felt uneasy about this report, since the language used was clearly drafted by the hospital lawyer in a manner seeking to justify the original action of suspension.

The last statement – "Dr. Fuentes's skillset is quite unique and beneficial to many patients" – was clearly in contradiction to the reason provided for his continued suspension, i.e., "might have posed a danger to any individual or the operation of the hospital."

The letter did not specify the factual basis that they were relying on in coming to this conclusion or, more generally, what was meant by this statement that had been extracted verbatim from the hospital by-laws.

The report's criticism of Dr. Fuentes for evaluating each complaint on its own merits was simply unacceptable for some members of the MEC. An older member of the MEC, Dr. Hoojin Kim, previously appointed chief of psychiatry, pointed out that if anything, rather than concluding that Dr. Fuentes is blameworthy for looking at each issue on its own facts, the report **should have evaluated whether the institution's complaint system was misused and weaponized by disgruntled individuals to gain** leverage and defame physicians.

He insisted "**Filing anonymous complaints to gain leverage is easy. Disproving them is harder, but what counts should be the facts underlying each matter rather than the existence of a complaint.**"

The insistence on the multiple incidents—and their "potential danger for patients or person's health or safety"—was clearly a desperate attempt by the lawyers to meet the burden required to label Dr. Fuentes behavior as disruptive (see: chapter 6).

Meanwhile, the reference to *"other specialties"* having challenges working with Dr. Fuentes was a disguised reference to cardiothoracic surgery, which was the *only* surgical specialty Dr. Fuentes had any issue interacting with, due to the ongoing competition between the cath lab's minimally invasive approach and the more invasive approach offered by cardiothoracic surgery.

Instead of recognizing the inability of cardiothoracic surgery to accept the progressive and minimally invasive procedures offered by Dr. Fuentes, the investigative committee focused instead on blaming him for every disagreement with them.

Interestingly, the four-person investigative committee declined to make any recommendations, leaving any such decision to the full MEC.

> *Although the Healthcare Quality Improvement Act may immunize hospitals and professional peer review bodies, those protections do not extend to peer reviews taken in bad faith or that do not conform with due process.*[40]

Once the investigative committee presented its investigation report to the MEC, a long discussion started.

Dr. Fuentes later heard from an undisclosed member of the MEC that the nurse union representative, Nurse Olivia Grogun, would not accept that no sanction was taken, and said that Dr. Fuentes **could not be brought back "just like that."** The nursing union's position led to another lengthy debate between the chairman of medicine, Dr. Friedland, and the union representative, Nurse Olivia Grogun, about reinstating Dr. Fuentes.

The medical staff president, Dr. Marie Rattner, recognized that they had a flimsy case against Dr. Fuentes and knew that if a vote was called to end Dr. Fuentes's suspension, the majority of the MEC members would probably vote to end it and reinstate him.

Dr. Marie Rattner was in a difficult spot. The nurse's union was pressuring her behind closed doors from the beginning to get rid of Dr. Fuentes, but the investigation didn't deliver what was required to do so.

---

40 https://sullivanlegal.us/hospital-may-be-liable-for-untrue-npdb-report/

On Nurse Union Power

One might wonder why the nurse unions are so strong. The ability of nurse unions to start a strike, paralyzing a hospital overnight, has given them tremendous leverage.[41] *This leverage has only gotten stronger with the growing number of nurses joining union ranks all over the country. And much of these union interests derived from the Covid-19 pandemic.*[42]

It should be noted that patient outcomes decline significantly during a nursing strike and the cost to the institution can be disastrous.[43]

At the same time, some hospitals have reported financial losses of over $40 million to train and replace nurses during large strikes while some others hospital had to close doors without ever being able to reopen.[44]

Other studies have shown that hospitals with unionized nurses might have slightly improved patient outcomes in the areas of hospital-acquired infections and readmission rates, but research is lacking for more specialized services such as interventional cardiology or specialized surgeries.[45]

---

41 NYC nurses strike and win historic contract https://www.nationalnursesunited.org/article/nyc-nurses-strike-and-win-historic-contract#:~:text=After%20a%20successful%20three%2Dday,employers%20fail%20to%20uphold%20contractual

42 https://time.com/5928528/frontline-workers-strikes-labor/

43 NURSE UNIONS AND PATIENT OUTCOMES ARINDRAJIT DUBE, ETHAN KAPLAN,ANDOWEN THOMPSON. ILRReview,69(4),August2016,pp.803–833 DOI:10.1177/0019793916644251

44 https://www.registerednursing.org/articles/do-unions-benefit-harm-healthcare-nursing/

45 https://www.registerednursing.org/articles/do-unions-benefit-harm-healthcare-nursing/

For institutions where nurses are not well-represented, or when overtime is too frequently requested, the union represents an attractive opportunity to create shared governance in the hospital as well as a stronger presence on several committees, including the medical executive committees and hospital boards.

In addition, unionized nurses have guaranteed pay raises and other benefits included in their contract. Nurse seniority is typically preferred to skill and knowledge, which goes hand in hand with a lack of performance-based incentives.

The direct consequence of unionization for the cath lab or the stroke unit, for instance, is the total lack of incentive for nurses to stay later or work harder, along with serious challenges to support highly specialized unionized nurses for any specialized service line.

In some institutions, the mandated wage increases and benefits packages are creating an unbearable cost. Nevertheless, one thing is clear: nurse unions are a big business, especially for their union leaders. Under the message of improving nurses' working conditions and patient outcomes, unions continue to advocate for their own survival first and foremost.[46]

As it became clear to Dr. Marie Rattner that the majority of the MEC was in favor of Dr. Fuentes's return, instead of calling for a vote to reinstate Dr. Fuentes, the medical staff president offered a compromise to recommend to Dr. Fuentes to attend a behavior assessment followed by a prompt return to his service.

46 https://www.registerednursing.org/articles/do-unions-benefit-harm-healthcare-nursing/

This recommendation was adopted unanimously by the MEC members, who it must be said, were tired of the lengthy meeting.

This deceiving maneuver allowed Dr. Rattner to delay Dr. Fuentes's return so that she could figure out her next move to prevent Dr. Fuentes's return.

Beyond the pressure from the nurse union, Dr. Marie Rattner always had animosity against Dr. Fuentes, ever since her arrival at the institution a few months prior. Trained as a geriatric physician, she was the exact opposite of Dr. Fuentes. While Dr. Fuentes was a charismatic and skilled academician, travelling the world and doing on-camera the most cutting-edge procedures in interventional cardiology, Dr. Rattner was confined to her private practice in the suburbs of Phoenix, seeing the same patients with blood pressures issues, constipation, and urinary incontinence. She had never travelled outside of Arizona and had never published or presented at any national meeting. She had always envied and despised Dr. Fuentes, who lived in a universe that she would never get to know now that she was a 65-year-old private physician, on the verge of retiring.

The Recommended Behavior Assessment

That same evening, Dr. Fuentes received a phone call from the chairman of medicine, Dr. Friedland, who recommended on behalf of the MEC that he attend the behavior assessment offered by the Professional Renewal Center in Kansas—or, if that wasn't available, then an alternative, similar course.

The next day, Dr. Fuentes attempted to register with the Professional Renewal Center (PRC) in Kansas but was told that it was not available for three months at least.[47]

Five days later, after several unanswered emails and phone calls to Mr. Ethan Sims, the medical staff director, Dr. Fuentes received a letter recommending him to attend PRC course.

The week before Dr. Fuentes received that letter, apparently, two behavior evaluation programs were discussed in an email chain among the chairman of medicine, the CMO, and the medical staff president, Dr. Marie Rattner: PRC and KSTAR. However, Dr. Fuentes was only offered PRC as an option.

The Truth about Physician Evaluation Programs and Remediation Programs

Historically, Physician Evaluation Programs (PEP) have provided a pathway for a physician addicted to alcohol or drugs to obtain the treatment necessary to return to the practice of medicine. PEPs have been very beneficial in this regard.

However, over the years, medical boards, state medical associations, and hospitals have developed exclusive relationships with "preferred" evaluation and treatment centers.

Neuropsychological testing was initially used to set a baseline of cognitive performance when an employee is being monitored for progression of disease or disability or to help differentiate between compromised cognition and stress-related cognitive complaints.

---

47 https://www.fsmb.org/siteassets/spex/pdfs/remedprog.pdf

Neuropsychological tests compare individuals' cognitive abilities to a normative standard, and their results can indicate impaired behavior that might compromise safety on the job. But using this type of testing to address behavioral or interpersonal issues doesn't make any sense, since those issues are best addressed by administrative or human resources interventions or through communication training.

Physician evaluation and treatment for alcohol, drug, mental, or behavioral problems has become a lucrative business. Indeed, the business model seems to be based on finding some type of pathology with physicians, who are deemed as having some deficit requiring some "remediation. Then, treatment centers recommend additional treatment at their center based on the evaluation performed at the same center. The remediation is typically expensive and time consuming. There are significant conflicts of interest.

Accusations of impairment, whether due to alcohol, drugs, mental or behavioral behavior, are accompanied by significant stigmatization. There is both self-stigmatization and external stigmatization by others. This stigmatization and moral damage that accompany false accusations can give rise to new psychopathologies that did not exist before (for example, anxiety or depression).

In addition, the assessment will place a blemish on the physician record, deepening the hole they are currently in since it can morph into restrictions or discipline with medical licensure, insurance contracts, and challenges with renewing professional liability insurance.

There are other entities that do behavioral assessments. In addition, there are private practitioners (board certified forensic psychiatrists) who have the same skill set and can perform an independent evaluation. The question is whether the hospital would accept any of these other individual or institutional evaluations.

The Recommendation of the MEC: Top 5 Takeaways

1. The investigative committee should perform a fair and diligent investigation in an unbiased manner and provide a recommendation at the end of the investigation.
2. The recommendation should be in alignment with the discovery of the investigation.
3. The legal team of the hospital should not be involved in the drafting of the investigative report.
4. Legal protections do not extend to peer reviews taken in bad faith or that do not conform with due process.
5. Be aware that physician evaluation programs could destroy your career and future ability to find a job, hence try to have them justify why you need to be assessed by one of those programs instead of by a forensic psychiatrist.

CHAPTER 8

THE COERCION

In the days following the presentation of the investigation report and the recommendation provided by the MEC, several key developments happened behind the scenes.

After the MEC deliberated extensively, as mentioned above, Dr. Friedland called Dr. Fuentes to let him know about the decision taken. He told him specifically that he needed to go in-person to the Professional Renewal Center (PRC) in Kansas. If this behavior assessment was not available within the next few weeks, Dr. Fuentes should find a similar course **so he could be reinstated as soon as possible.**

Dr. Fuentes was disappointed by the result and wanted to receive more information about the course. The following day he attempted to reach Mr. Ethan Sims, the Director of Medical Administration for that purpose without success. Instead, he received a letter advising him to participate in the Professional Renewal Center (PRC). The assessment is said to be completed over a four-day session on-site in Kansas. If Dr. Fuentes enrolled in the program, pertinent materials compiled by the MEC would be provided to the PCR and his permission would be needed to release a summary of their findings in a written report after the evaluation. The letter went on and claimed that this report will help the MEC decide how they can support his return to clinical activities.

The Coercion

After Dr. Fuentes contacted the PRC in Kansas and learned the behavior assessment's next available session was in three months, he again attempted to contact, without success, the Director of Medical Administration, Mr. Ethan Sims. At that time, he knew that Mr. Sims had also failed to get an earlier registration based on his discussion with the PRC team over the phone.

Confused and unable to get a reply from Mr. Sims, Dr. Fuentes tried to see if he could do a similar course earlier as suggested by Dr. Friedland. He identified another course in Nashville at Vanderbilt University—the Professional Development for Distressed Physician Behaviors course. He immediately registered.

The same day, in the evening, he received a phone call from Dr. Rattner explaining to him that in order to go to the PRC, **Dr. Fuentes would need to waive his hearing rights so that the recommendation of the MEC could be adopted by the board of the hospital**. More concerning was the fact that Dr. Rattner told him, "**No need to discuss this matter with your lawyer today, you are paying enough money as it is.**"

First thing in the morning the following day, Dr. Fuentes contacted his lawyer, Alan Rogers, who then demanded clarification from the hospital lawyer Dick Kosakov. Later that day Rogers received an email from the hospital lawyer, Mr. Kosakov **confirming the need for Dr. Fuentes to give up his hearing right in order**

for the recommendation from the MEC to go to the Hospital Board, who would allow him then to go to the PRC.

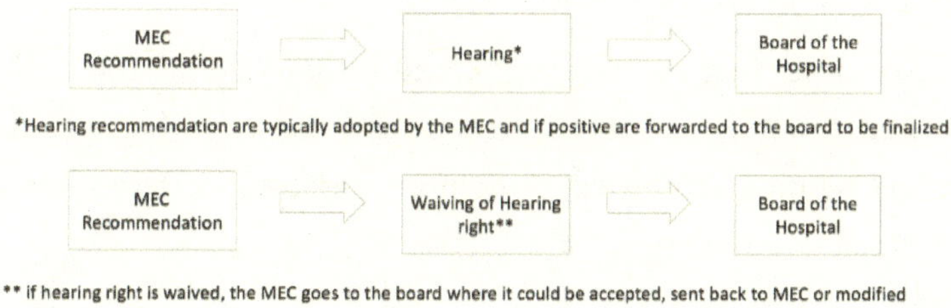

Pathway between MEC and board of the hospital and their relationship with the hearing.

Waive Your Hearing Rights?

A practitioner receiving an adverse action will be notified in writing accordingly. The notification will include the adverse action and the reasons for it. The practitioner will be provided with a right for a hearing. The hearing needs to be requested within the time frame required and, in the manner, specified (typically by certified mail).

The Practitioner may waive the right to a hearing by a signed statement submitted to the medical staff office or the CMO.

In the case of Dr. Fuentes, once he waives his right to a hearing, if the board of the hospital takes a negative action against him, he is left with only one recourse, an appeal process at the board level—but this is extremely limited because he would have accepted the recommendation of the MEC and all statements made against him up to that point. Hence it is recommended to only give up your hearing right if the hospital is offering you a settlement or if the hearing would not provide any benefit to your case, due to overwhelming evidence against you, for instance.

It became clear to Dr. Fuentes and his lawyer that the push to get him to waive his hearing rights was a coercion that would allow the hospital, if needed, to demote, sanction, or terminate Dr. Fuentes at a later date.

Indeed, if Dr. Fuentes gave up his hearing right, all documents and proofs accumulated until that point would be basically void. He wouldn't be able to challenge efficiently any sanction made by the hospital from this point on and would be left at the mercy of the hospital board in a final appeal.

> *If the action of the Board or MEC continues to be adverse to the practitioner, the Special Notice will inform the Practitioner of his or her right for an appeal at the Board of the hospital.*
>
> *The Hospital Board, may affirm, modify or reverse the adverse action. It could also refer the matter back to the MEC for further evaluation and modification. This entire process could take up to sixty days in duration.*

Behind the Scenes

What happened over the next few days was later exposed during the hearing at the hospital level.

After the MEC recommendation was provided to Dr. Fuentes by Dr. Friedland on behalf of the MEC, Dr. Mary Rattner kept being pressured by the nurse's union to make sure Dr. Fuentes did not come back. By then, even though the union knew that they didn't have a strong case against Dr. Fuentes, it wanted to protect their unionized nurses in the cath lab from the increasing workload and expertise requested from them under Dr. Fuentes's leadership. As explained (in chapter 6), the union favors seniority over expertise and at all cost the avoidance of overtime.

An email trail demonstrated that Dr. Friedland, Dr. Rattner, and Dr. Livingstone – **the day after** the MEC meeting – agreed to offer Dr. Fuentes either KSTAR (Knowledge, Skills, Training, Assessment and Research), available within a week in Texas, or PRC, available in three months at least. Instead of contacting Dr. Fuentes with that proposal, Dr. Rattner decided to impose on him the PRC, to delay his prompt return. But to be able to revoke his privileges, she needed to have his case moved directly to the medical board of the hospital, where Dr. Friedland, Dr. Fuentes's biggest supporter, didn't have a seat at the table and where the union would be well-represented.

Dr. Rattner called the hospital lawyer to ask for advice—he then created the basis for Dr. Fuentes's dilemma by binding his attendance to the behavior assessment on waiving his hearing right.

Indeed, since Dr. Fuentes hadn't exhausted all his remedies according to the hospital bylaws, the only way for his case to go to the board at this stage would be for him to give up his hearing right at the MEC level, moving directly the recommendation made to the board. Then the board could confirm or modify the recommendation made by the MEC—and more importantly make further recommendations including revocation of privileges.

Clearly the compromise that Dr. Friedland accepted from Dr. Rattner and the nurses' union was used against Dr. Fuentes. Not only did PRC became the only acceptable behavior assessment course, but in order to even go to PRC, Dr. Fuentes had to give up his hearing right.

The bottom line was that there was nothing justifying the MEC to recommend Dr. Fuentes to complete a behavior assessment course—and nothing justifying the unacceptable statement that Dr. Fuentes "*may pose a danger to any individual or the operation of the Hospital.*"

After discussing with his lawyer, Mr. Alan Rogers, Dr. Fuentes decided both to exercise his hearing right and to attend the Vanderbilt course in Nashville. It was imperative for Dr. Fuentes, who clearly didn't lack any fitness for duty, to demonstrate that he was trying to meet the MEC recommendation **while preserving his right to a hearing**. Moreover, since the NPDB was now available to all licensing boards, it became crucial to show his good faith in attending a course for destressed physicians, as long as he didn't give up his hearing rights.

The Coercion: Top 5 Takeaways

1. The by-laws of the hospital allow you to request a hearing and appeal any decision of the MEC.
2. Use every remedy provided to you by the hospital by-laws.
3. No practitioner should ever consider giving up his or her hearing right at the hospital level unless an acceptable settlement is offered.
4. Behavior assessments were tools initially utilized by hospitals to establish fitness for duty for physicians in rehabilitation. They've subsequently become used to seek any pathology (cognitive, psychiatric, or physical), justifying retroactively any actions taken against a physician.
5. Trust only official information provided in writing—any "informal" or "friendly" phone call by an administrative official has no legal weight in a court of law.

CHAPTER 9

THE HEARING

It is crucial for the practitioner wrongfully accused to request a hearing. The HCQIA requires it to take place before an independent hearing officer or review panel.[48] *You have the right to be represented by legal counsel, to receive a statement of all charges against you, to present your own proof, to call, examine, and cross-examine witnesses, and to have a record typed during the proceedings.*

> ***At the close of the hearing your attorney should submit a written statement, which should emphasize your core arguments and evidence. Ideally, making the case, you should propose that you receive no suspension at all and/or that the filing is voided at the NPDB altogether.***

48 Health Care Quality Improvement Act of 1986

For the reader to understand what a hearing at the hospital level looks like, one need to visualize the hearing very well-illustrated throughout the 2023 film *Oppenheimer*. **The hearing is not a trial, per se, but an internal tribunal working against the defendant. As in the movie, the burden of proof works against the defendant and there is no (or very little) discovery allowed.**

It took several months to set up Dr. Fuentes's hearing. First, the hospital attempted to hire as a hearing officer a lawyer who worked within their hospital systems. Dr. Fuentes's lawyer, Alan Rogers, was fast to object to that appointment and the hospital conceded.

Subsequently, another hearing officer with no personal involvement with the hospital was hired, but Dr. Fuentes's lawyer noticed that his firm represented the hospital in a prior case. This time, the objection of Dr. Fuentes's lawyer was ignored and the hospital pushed for appointing the hearing officer, Mr. Patrick Bauwen,

Perhaps at this point Dr. Fuentes's lawyer, Alan Rogers, should have sought an injunction from a judge to appoint an independent investigator, but Mr. Rogers did not, and they went forward, with Dr. Fuentes still in hopes for a fair hearing. Again, an experienced healthcare lawyer comfortable using state and federal law likely would've done otherwise, since the process at the hospital level is by definition biased against the practitioner.

The hearing officer (H.O.) started by asking for an introductory Zoom meeting to delineate the basic procedures during the hearing. He asked the hospital lawyer (Mr. Dick Kosakov) what he expected to achieve with the hearing, to which Mr. Kosakov responded that he didn't want to achieve anything. He just wanted to bring the H.O.'s recommendation back to the MEC.

The H.O. requested a written brief from each party. In their brief, the hospital lawyer intended to demonstrate at the hearing that the "*MEC's basis for action was reasonable and supported by the record. Due to the burden of proof against him, Dr. Fuentes would not be able to prevail.*"

Further the lawyer added, "*Dr. Fuentes's refusal to attend a behavior assessment will lead to termination of his privileges.*" **This statement was very problematic since Dr. Fuentes had to give up his hearing right prior to attending the required assessment course.**

The hearing is conducted according to rules of law relating to the examination of witnesses or presentation of evidence. ***However, any relevant evidence may be admitted by the H.O, regardless of the admissibility of such evidence in a court of law,*** *unless such evidence is deemed by the H.O. to be cumulative. Hearsay is admissible and shall be sufficient to support the decision of the H.O. The H.O may question witnesses or call additional witnesses if it deems appropriate.*

In all cases in which a hearing is conducted, after all the evidence has been submitted by both parties, ***the H.O. shall rule against the Practitioner*** *who requested the hearing unless he finds that such person has proved, by clear and convincing evidence, that the allegations against the Practitioner are untrue in total or in substantial part or unless it concludes, based on its findings of fact that the action of the MEC which prompted the hearing was arbitrary, unreasonable, or appears to be unfounded or unsupported by credible evidence.*

It is the burden of the Practitioner requesting the hearing to demonstrate that he satisfies, on a continuing basis, all

> *criteria for Clinical Privileges, and that he complies with all Medical Staff and Hospital policies.*
>
> *During the hearing, the Hospital may come forward initially with evidence in support of its decision. Thereafter, the burden shifts to the Practitioner who requested the hearing to come forward with evidence in his/her support.*

The Hearing Begins

The hospital lawyer called a total of 24 witnesses. As no nurses came forward, this required the hospital to subpoena nurses Simonar and Blevins.

To compensate the lack of nurses willing to come forward, the hospital lawyer called the director of personal, Ms. Clara Harari, and the HR representative who captured most complaints directed against Dr. Fuentes, Mr. Alan Troy.

The testimonies at the hearing, however, departed dramatically from the MEC report's conclusions and were far more derogatory towards Dr. Fuentes than anything set forth in the investigation report. It was clear the hospital lawyer, Mr. Dick Kosakov, was trying at all costs to meet the burden of proof of compromised patient safety by labeling Dr. Fuentes's behavior as disruptive. In other words, Dr. Fuentes was being punished for exercising his hearing right.

A member of the investigative committee, Dr. Stephanie Balley, testified at the hearing that the MEC investigative committee believed that **"there were some issues that we thought had a high probability of an adverse patient event."**

Some of his behaviors, the investigative committee felt, had a "high probability of delayed care and a high likelihood of an adverse event happening for the patient;" that certain staff were "afraid specifically of retaliation from Dr. Fuentes" and that based on Dr. Fuentes's conduct there was a "very high likelihood of a bad outcome for patients."

She further testified that this concern of a "very high likelihood of a bad outcome for patients" was shared "cumulatively" by the four-person investigative committee. But, ***none* of these alarmist conclusions or concerns were included *anywhere*** in the MEC Report.

It was extremely troubling to see the hospital witnesses at the hearing give testimony regarding Dr. Fuentes's conduct—and particularly Dr. Balley regarding how the investigative committee believed Dr. Fuentes to pose a threat to patients—without providing any concrete examples to support this testimony.

This significant discrepancy raised the strong inference that those testimonies alleging misbehavior by Dr. Fuentes were concocted at the hearing to justify retroactively the MEC's action in continuing Dr. Fuentes' suspension.

The fact that the hospital was now trying to use the hearing to reverse-engineer allegations against Dr. Fuentes that the investigative committee did not bother to include in its report provided a compelling basis for getting access to the interview notes taken by the investigative committee so it could be determined whether the allegations that got presented to the MEC had sound factual basis. Indeed, all interviews conducted by the investigative committee were captured and preserved but were not provided to Dr. Fuentes since limited discovery is allowed according to the bylaws.

Later, after weeks of debate between Dr. Fuentes's lawyer, Alan Rogers, and the hospital lawyer, Dick Kosakov, the hearing officer, Mr. Patrick Bauwen, forced the hospital attorney to provide the interview notes taken by the investigative committee.

It was astonishing to notice how much emphasis was placed on any negative testimonies while positive ones were summarized and incompletely integrated into the final report.

Moreover, most of these witnesses couldn't provide specific, concrete examples of unauthorized or improper interactions of Dr. Fuentes that would have had an adverse impact on patient care. Their testimony failed to meet the requirements that would allow for the suspension/revocation of hospital privileges. Instead, they all testified as to generalities in a conclusory way, which is precisely what courts reject as a basis for an adverse action against a physician's privileges.

> *The fact that a doctor ... has been 'unable to get along with' some doctors or hospital personnel is not a sufficient ground to exclude him from the use of hospitals... Physicians will not always agree as to the proper treatment for a patient or as to the proper practices in a hospital. The goal of providing high standards of medical care requires that physicians be permitted to assert their views when they feel that treatment of patients is improper or that negligent hospital practices are being followed. Considerations of harmony in the hospital must give way where the welfare of patients is involved, and a physician by making his objections known, whether or not tactfully done, should not be required to risk his right to practice medicine. Moreover, a hospital district should not be permitted to adopt standards*

> *for the exclusion of doctors from the use of its hospital which are so vague and ambiguous as to provide a substantial danger of arbitrary discrimination in their application. In asserting their views as to proper treatment and hospital practices, many physicians will become involved in a certain amount of dispute and friction, and a determination that such common occurrences have more than their usual significance and show temperamental unsuitability for hospital practice of one of the doctors is of necessity highly conjectural. In these circumstances there is a danger that the requirement of temperamental suitability will be applied as a subterfuge where considerations having no relevance to fitness are present.*[49]

"Testimony," AKA Manufactured Falsehood

During the hearing, the medical staff's president, Dr. Rattner, testified that the events summarized in the perfect storm chapter, justified the suspension. Dr. Fuentes allegedly interfered with the resuscitation of a patient who had had a cardiac arrest, and later Dr. Fuentes demanded an intubated patient to be brought to the cath lab, while behaving with hostility, anger, shouting, and aggressive behavior.

First, Dr. Fuentes in no way interfered with the resuscitation of the patient who had coded. As recounted by Dr. Rafael Sabatini,

---

49 Rosner v Eden Twp. Hosp. Dist., 58 Cal 2d 592, 598, 375 P2d 431, 434-35 [1962], cited with approval by Miller v Eisenhower Med. Ctr., 27 Cal 3d 614, 629, 614 P2d 258, 267 [1980], cited with approval by Nanavati v Burdette Tomlin Mem. Hosp., 107 NJ 240, 253, 526 A2d 697, 704 [1987].

the anesthesiologist in the unit that day, nothing about the morning conversation (as captured on a soundless security video) was inappropriate. Dr. Fuentes did nothing to interfere with this code, contrary to the second-hand and false information that had been conveyed to Dr. Rattner by the chief medical officer, Dr. Livingstone, and/or Mrs. Clara Harari, the director of personnel.

Second, Dr. Fuentes did not want an intubated patient brought to the cath lab. In fact, nurse Jane Clark had called for an intubated patient in error and Dr. Fuentes told her he wanted a non-intubated patient. Nurse Jane Clark's story at the hearing was contradicted and refuted by her statement to the HR representative Mr. Alan Troy and also the sign-out sheets for the day proving that the intubated patient was never brought down to the unit.

Third, nurse Simonar claimed that Dr. Fuentes "yelled" at nurse Clark, who even filed a workplace violence "claim" to support his allegation, citing that Dr. Fuentes "verbally assaulted" nurse Clark. However, nurse Clark repeatedly denied that Dr. Fuentes yelled at him. Dr. Grant investigated and wrote in his report of nurse Simonar claim that there was no yelling or workplace violence.

The Hospital also failed to call the four other witnesses (besides nurse Clark) who nurse Simonar identified as witnesses to the yelling incident.

Thus, the main allegation that the hospital used to initially suspend Dr. Fuentes **never happened!**

The hospital lawyer also relied on Dr. Stephanie Balley (one of four-member investigative committee) to claim that there was a high likelihood of Dr. Fuentes causing an adverse patient event. The only concrete example he offered for this conclusion was Dr. Fuentes's supposed interference with Dr. Janet Brauer, the cardiothoracic surgeon performing a thoracotomy on a patient during a cardiologic intervention complicated by a cardiovascular arrest.

Neither this example nor conclusion were included in the report, and neither were corroborated with any documentation, whatsoever. Moreover, three doctors who were present during the entire procedure as well as two technicians all denied under oath in this hearing that Dr. Fuentes interfered with Dr. Brauer performing the thoracotomy. The hospital also failed to call to testify any anesthesiologist who Dr. Brauer claimed Dr. Fuentes was arguing with and causing her to delay starting the thoracotomy. Dr. Brauer claimed Dr. Sabatini was a witness to this alleged argument, but Dr. Sabatini's testimony directly refuted her testimony. Dr. Sabatini testified that there was no delay in connection with Dr. Brauer's efforts to resuscitate the patient. Dr. Sabatini even pointed out that Dr. Fuentes helped the anesthesia team in the resuscitation of the patient by placing a central venous access during the code to assess the venous pressure appropriately.

The most obvious conclusion from Dr. Brauer's totally uncorroborated story is that she fabricated the claim that Dr. Fuentes caused her to delay the thoracotomy procedure. She had several strong motives to have lied, including (A) as reflected in the interview notes, that she was blamed for the patient's death because it "took too long to cut into the [patient's chest]" and (B) she harbored a racist animus towards Dr. Fuentes, which was manifested by her mocking of Dr. Fuentes's accent, as witnessed by one of Dr. Fuentes's nurses.

Thus, two of the most significant events that the hospital relied on to justify its actions were manufactured falsehoods. In an analogous context, when employment discrimination is at issue,

> In appropriate circumstances, the trier of fact can reasonably infer from the falsity of the explanation that the employer is dissembling to cover up

> a discriminatory purpose. Such an inference is consistent with the general principle of evidence law that the factfinder is entitled to consider a party's dishonesty about a material fact as "affirmative evidence of guilt.[50]

Here, we should conclude that the hospital relied on impermissible considerations when it acted to continue the suspension of Dr. Fuentes's hospital privileges.

Based on the aforementioned, Dr. Fuentes met his burden under the hospital by-laws and proved, by clear and convincing evidence,[51] that the factual allegations against him were untrue in total or in substantial part, and/or the evidence supports a finding that the MEC decision to suspend and/or revoke his privileges was arbitrary, unreasonable, and unsupported by credible evidence.[52]

The hospital by-laws must also be read in conjunction with state law governing the circumstances called the Nanavati standard, when a hospital may revoke a doctor's hospital privileges, which provides:

---

50 Reeves v Sanderson Plumbing Products, Inc., 530 US 133, 147-48, 120 S Ct 2097, 2108-09, 147 L Ed 2d 105 [2000].

51 *See* In re Samay, 166 NJ 25, 30, 764 A2d 398, 401 [2001]("Clear and convincing evidence is that which produce[s] in the mind of the trier of fact a firm belief or conviction as to the truth of the allegations sought to be established, evidence so clear, direct and weighty and convincing as to enable (the factfinder) to come to a clear conviction, without hesitancy, of the truth of the precise facts in issue.")(Internal quotations omitted).

52 The Hospital in its Pre-Hearing Brief argued both that "This matter involves a precautionary suspension of Dr. Fuentes, which was ultimately continued pending Dr. Fuentes's participation in an approved comprehensive assessment program, and that Dr. Fuentes's failure to attend an approved assessment course makes him ineligible for continued privileges. It thus appears that the Hospital has in suspended, and also *de facto* revoked, his privileges because he did not attend PRC, which he could only have done had he first waived his hearing rights.

Doctors, like other people, have quirks, and some doctors are more disagreeable than others. The mere fact that a doctor is irascible, however, does not constitute good cause for termination of his or her hospital privileges. Nor should allegations of "disharmony" ever be used as a ruse to deny or terminate staff privileges because of a doctor's race, religion, color, or gender. Likewise, a doctor should not be cut off from staff membership merely because he or she has criticized hospital practices and other doctors. When a doctor's conduct actually interferes with patient care, the disruption justifies ending his or her privileges. For disharmony to constitute good cause for dismissal from a hospital staff, however, it is unnecessary that it cause actual harm to patients. Nonetheless, more should be required than general complaints of a physician's inability to cooperate with others. To constitute disruptive behavior meriting termination of staff privileges, hospital authorities should present concrete evidence of specific instances of misbehavior, such as unjustified altercations with other doctors or nurses, violations of hospital routines or rules, breaches of professional standards, or the commission of some other act that will adversely affect health care delivery. In setting the appropriate standard for denial or revocation of a doctor's privileges, we return to the premise that a decision concerning those privileges affects the hospital, the doctor, and his or her patients. We believe we strike the appropriate balance by requiring that the hospital establish that prospective disharmony will probably have an adverse impact on patient care. The mere fact that the doctor annoys other doctors, nurses, and administrators is insufficient. A doctor may be so disruptive, however, as to throw the hospital into turmoil and prevent it from functioning effectively. So substantial a disruption could lead the hospital authorities to conclude that the probable outcome will be harm to the patients.[53]

Under state law, application of anything less than what is required under the ***Nanavati Standard*** constitutes a denial of a physician's right to a "fair hearing."[54]

After the investigation, when the hospital continued the suspension of Dr. Fuentes's privileges, neither the report nor the hospital letter (later sent to Dr. Fuentes, advising him of his continued his suspension) reflected that any "prospective disharmony [between him and others at the hospital] will probably have an adverse impact on patient care."[55] That is, at the time of his suspension, and

---

53 Nanavati v Burdette Tomlin Mem. Hosp., 107 NJ 240, 253, 526 A2d 697, 704 [1987] (internal quotations and citations omitted) (the "Nanavati Standard").

54 Nanavati v Cape Regional Med. Ctr., A-4111-17T3, 2020 WL 2529523, at *5 [NJ Super Ct App Div May 19, 2020] ("Application of a less exacting standard [than Nanavati] for [the doctor's] conduct to impact patient care prejudiced his right to a fair hearing.").

55 Some hospitals enact specific by-laws that provide "that the disruptive conduct of a physician, in the sense of his or her inability to work in harmony with other health care personnel at the hospital, is a ground for denying, suspending, restricting, refusing to renew or revoking the staff appointment or clinical privileges of the offending physician, when such inability may have an adverse impact upon overall patient care at the hospital." *See* Mahmoodian v United Hosp. Ctr., Inc., 185 W Va 59, 69, 404

even in its pre-hearing brief, the hospital lawyer failed to articulate a basis for the suspension or revocation of privileges that met the controlling **Nanavati Standard**.

Instead, the hospital shifted its position, and only began arguing during the hearing that Dr. Fuentes's conduct could have had an adverse effect on patient care, initially via the testimony of Dr. Stephanie Balley, one of the four-member investigative committee. The fact that the report omitted any such conclusion should be viewed as a deliberate determination by the hospital that, following the investigation (which included interviewing 18 witnesses and reviewing many documents), there was no basis under the Nanavati Standard to revoke or suspend Dr. Fuentes' privileges.

Although the report had four signatories, Dr. Stephanie Balley was the only signatory whom the hospital called to testify. There is no evidence that any of the other three signatories to the report agreed with Dr. Stephanie Balley's testimony to the extent it goes beyond what's contained in the report. One can only conclude, because the hospital lawyer did not call those doctors to testify, that those individuals do not agree with anything Dr. Balley testified about beyond what's written in the report.[56]

SE2d 750, 760 [1991]. Any Hospital By-Laws is constrained to meet the Nanavati Standard.

56 Such an uncalled witness inference is appropriate where: (1) that the uncalled witness is peculiarly within the control or power of only the one party, or that there is a special relationship between the party and the witness or the party has superior knowledge of the identity of the witness or of the testimony the witness might be expected to give; (2) that the witness is available to that party both practically and physically; (3) that the testimony of the uncalled witness will elucidate relevant and critical facts in issue [;] and (4) that such testimony appears to be superior to that already utilized in respect to the fact to be proven. State v Hill, 199 NJ 545, 561, 974 A2d 403, 413 [2009].

Moreover, the hospital failed to sustain its burden under the Nanavati Standard of "present[ing] concrete evidence of specific instances of misbehavior, such as unjustified altercations with other doctors or nurses, violations of hospital routines or rules, breaches of professional standards, or the commission of some other act that will adversely affect health care delivery."

But what are the facts demonstrated at the end of the hearing?

Dr. Fuentes is a world renowned and highly experienced interventional cardiologist with nearly 400 published papers to his name and over 20 years of experience working in the field. He is invited to hospitals internationally to train doctors in his specialty. Doctors from around the world have also come to train under his guidance. He was hired to build a world class interventional cardiology program that was anticipated to treat a large number of patients. The hospital report recognized that, "All parties interviewed agreed that he offers a unique skill set that would be difficult to replace and offers clinical expertise that benefits a particular patient population."

He ran into resistance in building the department on two fronts (at least) from the outset of his employment. As Dr. Sabatini testified, many anesthesiologists did not view working in the cath lab as desirable due to the high volume of cases that they would be required to work on as compared to other services. According to Dr. Sabatini, this created "tension between the two services as increased demand in the cath lab created increased demand from anesthesia services, which they were not able to meet in a timely fashion," per Dr. Sabatini's testimony. That tension was ultimately resolved, as Dr. Romeo Sabatini acknowledged, by selecting anesthesiologists interested in working in the cath lab.

As cath lab technician Sam Santori also testified, a number of nurses were unhappy working in a fast paced, high-volume department when previously the cath lab had been viewed by nurses as a cushy, slow-paced, and relatively easy place to work.

Despite the hospital's aggressive efforts to paint Dr. Fuentes as a disruptive physician who presented a danger to patients, the exact opposite was the case, as confirmed by the testimony of Dr. Grant, who testified that Dr. Fuentes completely prioritizes patient safety and insisted that no nurse had come to him with a safety concern.

Dr. Grant's testimony is especially noteworthy, because not even Dr. Fuentes's superior, who bears responsibility for what happens in the department of cardiology and obviously has a vested interest in ensuring the safety of the patients in the department of the hospital over which he had responsibility; he also did not agree with the hospital position at the hearing that Dr. Fuentes posed a danger to patients. It's unfathomable that Dr. Grant would permit Dr. Fuentes to continue working in his department if he had even a scintilla of doubt regarding patient safety being at risk on account of Dr. Fuentes's conduct.

Dr. Grant's opinion that Dr. Fuentes prioritized patient care and safety was shared at the hearing by twenty-two witnesses with direct knowledge of his behavior and who interacted with him on a regular basis. They testified under oath that Dr. Fuentes is someone who prioritized patient care, was a fierce patient advocate, and treated with dignity and respect the people who worked with and around him. An anesthesiologist also told the investigative committee that "Dr. Fuentes challenges recommendations and can be 'pushy' but ultimately concedes to recommendations from anesthesia. Notes that he has not felt unduly pressured to adjust practice or recommendations."

Another fact: Dr. Fuentes was willing to attend an approved behavioral assessment. In its pre-hearing brief, the hospital justified its decision to suspend Dr. Fuentes's privileges (in part) because, "Dr. Fuentes's actions in failing to attend the recommended behavioral assessment and unilaterally deciding to choose his own course further demonstrates his poor collaboration with the hospital" and concluded that his "failure to attend an approved assessment course makes him susceptible to lose his privileges."

However, the evidence established that Dr. Fuentes was willing to attend the approved behavioral assessment program, but it was unavailable for the next three months (something the medical staff knew at the time it told him about it). He thus asked for permission to attend a program at Vanderbilt University, but was told by Dr. Rattner that the Nashville program did not meet the hospital's standards and that he could "do better."

In fact, Dr. Rattner had approved, in an email, for Dr. Fuentes an alternative program, KSTAR, that was available within a few weeks, after it was recommended by Mr. Sims. The hospital, however, unjustifiably concealed this program from Dr. Fuentes because Mrs. Laura Browning, the hospital CEO, overruled Dr. Rattner's decision to offer the alternative program to Dr. Fuentes, despite her status as a non-voting member of the medicals staff, based on her untested belief that the hospital's board would not approve it, despite knowing nothing about it.

Mr. Sims's email recommending KSTAR indicated that both programs "would issue a 'fitness for duty'... one just puts more burden on the hospital to determine next steps." The hospital unjustifiably chose to delay the process that could result in the reinstatement of his privileges.

Dr. Fuentes, having no other options, attended at his own expense the program in Nashville while on suspension and provided the results to the medical staff, hoping that said results might persuade the medical staff to reconsider. Instead, the medical staff's counsel faulted him for taking an unapproved course. Of course, this wouldn't have happened had the medical staff disclosed to Dr. Fuentes that it had approved the alternative program, which was available at around the same time as the Nashville program.

Moreover, as the hospital and its outside counsel made clear to Dr. Fuentes, the Board of Directors would not approve the recommendation that he attend a behavioral assessment program unless he first waived his hearing rights. Thus, the hospital, by concluding in its pre-hearing brief that Dr. Fuentes's "failure to attend an approved assessment course makes him ineligible for continued privileges," retaliated against him for invoking his contractual Fair Hearing rights under the by-laws.

In an email, Dr. Fuentes's lawyer, Alan Rogers, asked if his client has a right to a hearing/appeal after completing the course/assessment if adverse action is taken against him. To which the hospital lawyer made it clear that no hearing at the MEC level would be possible once Dr. Fuentes waived his hearing right.

Thus, it would have been a "fool's errand" for Dr. Fuentes to have waived his Fair Hearing rights and then expected the hospital to grant him a fair hearing if things did not turn out his way. Surely, with a signed waiver in hand, the hospital would have been fully justified under the by-laws in denying him a fair hearing, especially when coupled with the clear statement from its counsel.

Thus, Dr. Fuentes had the Hobson's Choice of pursing his contractual Fair Hearing rights under the by-laws or waiving them as a pre-condition of the Board of Directors considering the hospital recommendation that he attend an assessment program. In the hearing, Dr. Fuentes was now being punished through the suspension of his privileges for exercising his right, thus establishing that the hospital decision that Dr. Fuentes was not eligible for continued privileges was arbitrary and/or unreasonable and contrary to state law that prohibits "retaliation… based on the employee's exercise of certain established rights, violating a clear mandate of public policy."[57]

Under state and federal law, Dr. Fuentes has the right to a hearing and judicial review flowing from that hearing if his hospital privileges are suspended or revoked. The hospital had punished him for invoking that fundamental right to a hearing embedded in the state law.[58]

Many other irregularities prejudicially tainted the hospital's actions against Dr. Fuentes.

- The personal director Ms. Clara Harari admitted that she lost her notes of her presentation made to the medical staff during the initial hearing of Dr. Fuentes with the MEC (Chapter 4). Mr. Troy testified that any disappearance of notes would have been entirely improper for an HR department. Mr. Sims also admitted that he destroyed his notes of the meeting. This destruction of key evidence warrants an adverse inference for

---

57 MacDougall v Weichert, 144 NJ 380, 393, 677 A2d 162, 168 [1996].

58 See Nanavati, supra; Garrow v Elizabeth Gen. Hosp. and Dispensary, 79 NJ 549, 557, 401 A2d 533, 537 [1979]; Hernandez v Overlook Hosp., 149 NJ 68, 692 A2d 971 [1997].

spoliation of evidence.[59]

- Human Resources also omitted from its Executive Summary of the investigation of the "perfect storm" events that was provided to the hospital the admissions of nurse Clark that exonerated Dr. Fuentes of the accusations that he "yelled" at Clark and had asked for an intubated patient to be brought to the cath lab, thus concealing key exculpatory evidence from the medical staff.
- Nurse Blevins admitted that his Workplace Conduct Incident Report contained a false allegation that Dr. Fuentes took a video of staff, yet the hospital continues to rely on his allegations to sustain its case against him.
- Mr. Sims and/or Dr. Rattner failed to disclose to the hospital Dr. Grant's reports of his three investigations of claims filed, thus concealing pertinent information that may well have affected the final decision-making process.
- Mr. Sims also admitted that he failed to supply to the investigative committee the interview notes of an interview that were highly supportive of Dr. Fuentes from an oncologic surgeon. Interestingly he testified that he never had issues working with Dr. Fuentes even when there was a difference of opinion, that patient care was never affected, and that he never observed unprofessional behavior towards staff. He did however voice a concern about the impact of losing such "an innovative, cutting-edge talent."

---

59 Dr. Fuentes testified that Mrs. Harari accused him falsely on August 24, 2022, when presenting the hospital position to the Medical Staff, of performing procedures on patients without their approval. Mrs. Harari claimed a lack of recollection of what she said to the Medical Staff. Conveniently for her, her memory could not be refreshed because she lost his notes of what she said.

While Mr. Sims claims his omission was an oversight, this explanation isn't worthy of credence considering that the interview notes omitted directly undermined the very grounds upon which the Hospital sought to criticize Dr. Fuentes, and that Mr. Sims worked closely with hospital's counsel in preparing the report.

Indeed, Mr. Sims, in drafting the report, also twisted one nurse's interview statement to the investigative committee that there was not an "us vs them" culture in the cath lab to the completely opposite statement that "the committee has identified that the ongoing communication challenges presented regarding Dr. Fuentes have promulgated "a culture of 'us' vs. 'them' in regards to relationships between the interventional cardiologists and other members of the multi-disciplinary care team, specifically in reference to the nursing staff within the cath lab."

Taken as a whole, the entire process had been tainted by the hospital's disregard for the truth surrounding Dr. Fuentes. Had the hospital thought Dr. Fuentes was a threat to patient safety, it would have revoked his privileges after the report was issued. Instead, the medical staff sought to coerce Dr. Fuentes into waiving his hearing rights so that it could have taken whatever action it wanted without having to address the extensive record that supports Dr. Fuentes that had been presented in this case.

The Hearing: Top 5 Takeaways

1. During the hearing, the burden of proof works against the physician, and there is no (or very little) discovery allowed.
2. Hearsay is permissible and can be used to incriminate the practitioner.

3. The hospital will find and proctor people antagonistic to the practitioner to testify.
4. In some cases the hearing officer, paid by the hospital, will act as both a judge and a jury, making the process even more biased.
5. It is exceptional for the practitioner to prevail if a hearing is not following state of federal laws.

CHAPTER 10

LEGAL ANALYSIS OF THE HEARING FACTS

The following is a legal analysis of the hearing facts established by Dr. Fuentes's legal team.

1. The Perfect Storm Event

One of the key witnesses on that day was nurse Christopher Simonar. In his testimony, he contradicted nurse Jane Clark (the alleged victim of the "verbal assault"), who made clear that Dr. Fuentes had not yelled at her, and his own statement to Dr. Grant that stated Dr. Fuentes had not yelled at nurse Clark. He also testified that he spoke with nurse Clark before he filed her claim, which nurse Clark confirmed in her testimony. He was well aware that there was no yelling, yet he filed a verge that falsely accused Dr. Fuentes of yelling, thus showing a malicious intent, as his claim was based on a total falsehood.

Moreover, nurse Simonar had decided to leave the institution after having been criticized for his poor performance over a long period by Dr. Fuentes and the other physicians working in the cath lab, and thus he had a strong motive on the day of his resignation to retaliate against Dr. Fuentes.

Dr. Grant concluded that nurse Simonar "us[ed] threats to harm the reputations of the physicians, such as claiming violence, when in this case there was none" in order to gain leverage in working out differences. Despite Dr. Grant's clear rejection of nurse Simonar's false allegation, the hospital has perversely seized on it as a primary justification for suspending Dr. Fuentes' privileges *a month* after the perfect storm event.

Nurse Simonar also evidenced a significant animus towards Dr. Fuentes, including by calling the HR representative Mr. Alan Troy after he left the hospital to report falsely that he had told him to cover up an incident where a colleague of Dr. Fuentes had cursed at him. In fact, Dr. Fuentes did the opposite and had directed that colleague to apologize to him, as confirmed by text messages between Dr. Fuentes and nurse Blevins and an email in which he directed his colleague to write and send an apology letter for his conduct towards nurse Simonar. In his testimony, nurse Simonar denied calling Mr. Troy, but Mr. Troy's notes and testimony reflect otherwise. Nurse Simonar acknowledged grudgingly in his hearing testimony that the colleague apologized to him, but then denigrated his apology.

Nurse Simonar is thus particularly not credible, especially when factoring that a subpoena was issued to bring him to testify.

Thus, there is no evidence to support the alleged "verbal assault" other than nurse Simonar's completely discredited account. We should also conclude that the hospital chose not to call any of the witnesses nurse Simonar identified in his claim as witnesses to the alleged "verbal assault" because none of them would corroborate it, especially considering that nurse Clark, as the alleged victim, denied that it happened.

Nurse Blevins, meanwhile, also testified that Dr. Fuentes "yelled" at nurse Clark. This testimony was based obviously on what he heard from someone else (not nurse Clark), since he was on vacation. This assertion, which is clearly not true, coupled with his admission that he filed a false complaint accusing Dr. Fuentes of taking a video of staff, totally undermines his credibility and any of his allegations that Dr. Fuentes was yelling at staff and him on a regular basis. If such yelling was going on one would expect that someone other than nurse Simonar would corroborate it. However, nobody else did.

Moreover, Mrs. Harari, who presented the hospital position to the medical staff on at the request of the CEO and/or CMO, lost her notes of her presentation (which she shared with the hospital's counsel before her presentation) immediately after the meeting and failed to save those notes on her computer. Likewise, Mr. Sims, who took contemporaneous notes of the meeting also destroyed his notes. This destruction of evidence constitutes spoliation of evidence, and probably both their notes contained information favorable to Dr. Fuentes that undermine the hospital decision to suspend Dr. Fuentes's privileges.[60]

---

60 Izzo v Off. of Regulatory Affairs, A-0462-21, 2023 WL 4055649, at *4 [NJ Super Ct App Div June 19, 2023]("A spoliation inference may be drawn when an ALJ finds it appropriate to "infer that the evidence destroyed or concealed would not have been favorable to the spoliator" and such inference serves to "even[ ] the playing field where evidence has been hidden or destroyed.").

2. The Percutaneous Transluminal Coronarography Angioplasty (PTCA)

The Hospital relied heavily on an alleged incident that occurred a year prior in connection with a PTCA performed on a patient by Dr. Fuentes. Dr. Stephanie Balley identified only one concrete incident that allegedly left her with the view that there was a high likelihood of an adverse patient event occurring were Dr. Fuentes's privileges not suspended. That event was Dr. Fuentes allegedly interfering with Dr. Janet Brauer performing a thoracotomy on the patient who had coded during the PTCA procedure. As Dr. Stephanie Balley admitted, this alleged incident of interference was not recounted in the report or in the notes of the subcommittee's interview with Dr. Brauer. It is also not mentioned in the hospital lawyer's pre-hearing brief.

The hospital has not offered a shred of documentary proof to corroborate this alleged incident (not a claim, not an operative report, not a memorandum to file, nothing at all). Dr. Stephanie Balley's version is based on what she says Dr. Brauer told her (since she was not present when the incident allegedly happened), to the effect that Dr. Fuentes interfered with Dr. Brauer performing the procedure. Dr. Brauer claimed, in a different version of what happened, that she waited to do anything to help the patient while Dr. Fuentes was engaged in an "unfathomable" argument with one or more anesthesiologists, whose names she couldn't fully recall.

Against this extreme paucity of evidence, all other witnesses present denied that Dr. Fuentes did anything to interfere with or delay Dr. Brauer from performing the thoracotomy. As noted above, Dr. Sabatini, the anesthesiologist on the case, testified that there was no delay in Dr. Brauer taking lifesaving measures for the patient.

The hospital also failed to call to testify, or even identify, all the anesthesiologist(s) with whom Dr. Fuentes was supposedly arguing.

Dr. Rattner testified that she had heard about an issue arising in connection with the PTCA procedure, which was that an unnamed anesthesiologist thought there was a problem and Dr. Fuentes supposedly did not. Although this supposedly concerned her and she spoke with Dr. Friedland about it, she did nothing further, and the matter never came before the Medical Executive Committee. Dr. Rattner said nothing in her testimony about Dr. Fuentes interfering with Dr. Brauer performing a lifesaving procedure on a patient, further undermining Dr. Brauer's claim.

We should draw the inference that Dr. Brauer fabricated the story from the fact that no anesthesiologist who was present during the PTCA procedure was called by the hospital to testify, along with and the rest of the evidence. For such a significant allegation in connection with a procedure for which there was a root cause analysis (RCA), a morbidity and mortality meeting (M&M), and a report to the Department of Health, one would expect there to be at least some corroborating proof that Dr. Fuentes had interfered with Dr. Brauer taking lifesaving measures. Yet nothing whatsoever has been produced.

Dr. Brauer, however, who harbored a racist attitude towards Dr. Fuentes as evidenced by her mocking of Dr. Fuentes' accent, had a significant motive to fabricate the story, because she chafed at the fact, as reflected in the subcommittee's interview notes, that "blame was shifted to anesthesia and cardiothoracic surgery" (took too long to cut into chest to perform thoracotomy). That is, she was blamed for an adverse patient outcome in a procedure that Dr. Fuentes started. Dr. Brauer's false allegation against Dr. Fuentes in connection with the PTCA procedure constitutes defamation and a violation of the AMA's Code of Ethics: "Physicians must not submit false or malicious reports of disruptive behavior."

The hospital has misused the unfortunate events surrounding the PTCA patient to argue that Dr. Fuentes's behavior in the procedure would result in harm to patients. However, other than Dr. Brauer's uncorroborated, vague, and unsupported version, all the evidence supports the conclusion that Dr. Brauer's story was pure fiction, which she made-up to exact retribution against Dr. Fuentes, and should not serve as a basis to revoke Dr. Fuentes's hospital privileges.

3. The Valve Situation

Dr. Ralph Liota filed two claims against Dr. Fuentes involving a patient of his who Dr. Liota, without consulting him, decided needed invasive and dangerous cardiac exploratory surgery including a thoracotomy that could have permanently maimed the patient. Dr. Fuentes had placed a valve in the patient's heart during a minimally invasively procedure the prior day. The patient developed a partial blockage and came back to the hospital's ICU the next day. Once Dr. Fuentes was alerted that his patient was in the ICU, he came to bring his patient to the cath lab so he could readjust the valve. He consulted with Dr. Marc Reely, a general surgeon, in his role as the mediator between the cardiology service and the cardiothoracic surgery service, and he concurred that this was the correct way to proceed, especially since the patient had been initially admitted on his service. Dr. Fuentes's colleague, Bruce Waine, readjusted the valve in a short, minimally invasive procedure and the patient recovered well.

Nonetheless, Dr. Liota filed two claims, describing that Dr. Fuentes had interacted with him in an unprofessional way. Dr. Grant was appointed to investigate his claim, and he prepared a report following his investigation that cleared Dr. Fuentes of any wrongdoing. He also confirmed in his testimony that Dr. Fuentes did nothing wrong, nor did he jeopardize patient safety, in connection with the situation involving Dr. Liota. Witnesses to the interaction between Dr. Fuentes and Dr. Liota also testified at the hearing that Dr. Fuentes acted professionally in his interaction with Dr. Liota.

One of the witnesses opined that Dr. Fuentes helped prevent a malpractice case by ensuring that the patient did not get operated on by Dr. Liota, which could have resulted in the patient experiencing severe morbidity form thoracotomy that Dr. Liota wanted to perform. Dr. Fuentes's conduct in advocating forcefully for his patient is fully consistent with the AMA Code of Ethics and the Nanavati Standard and was confirmed by Dr. Grant in his report on Dr. Liota's verges.

Inexplicably, the hospital was never provided with Dr. Grant's investigation report of Dr. Liota's verges, which was mysteriously only produced on the eve of Dr. Grant testifying in this case and which delayed his testimony.

While the hospital claims that Dr. Grant was at fault for not submitting his report correctly on the hospital internal digital claim system, even a minimal investigation by the hospital (such as an interview with Dr. Grant or with Dr. Liota, who acknowledged being interviewed by Dr. Grant) would have revealed that the former investigated and filed a report rejecting Dr. Liota's claims. In fact, one of his complaints indicated the "hospital physician leadership to provide follow up." Thus, the hospital, which was provided with Dr. Liota's verges, should have tracked down the follow-up to the claim rather than feign surprise and blame Dr. Grant for misfiling his report, which in any event he emailed to HR, Dr. Rattner, and Dr. Friedland. This is another instance of willful ignorance, this time by the hospital, in not tracking down Dr. Grant's report on Dr. Liota's verges, especially because the hospital relied on Dr. Liota's claims in suspending Dr. Fuentes's privileges.

4. The Unstable Coronary Unit Patient

Three years prior, nurse Patrick Noah filed a claim against Dr. Fuentes concerning an incident that allegedly happened between Dr. Fuentes and Dr. Brauer in the patient's room in the CCU. A senior executive nurse was tasked with investigating the claim, but there was no close-out of the claim and no written report had been produced, suggesting strongly that the matter was not viewed as problematic.

The situation involved a patient who had been admitted to Dr. Fuentes's service but who was brough to the CCU because he was extremely sick. Dr. Brauer unilaterally and without consulting Dr. Fuentes decided the patient should have surgery. Dr. Fuentes was called to the CCU, where he proceeded to have a discussion with Dr. Brauer about whether the patient needed surgery. The patient was comatose and could not hear the discussion. The entire interaction between Dr. Brauer and Dr. Fuentes was witnessed by Dr. Romanov, the coronary unit cardiologist, who testified at length that Dr. Fuentes acted firmly but professionally in his interaction with Dr. Brauer, especially because the matter involved the patient's life. Dr. Romanov directly refuted nurse Noah and Dr. Brauer's claims that Dr. Fuentes acted improperly in the patient's room.

Dr. Fuentes persuaded Dr. Brauer and her supervisor Dr. Mark Salmon to allow him to perform a percutaneous transluminal coronarography to establish that the patient did not need invasive surgery. Dr. Fuentes started his procedure on the patient, which took around 10 minutes, and was then evicted from the angiography room by Dr. Brauer even though the procedure that he performed established that there was no coronary obstruction.

Dr. Rafael Navin, the previous CMO, testified that this situation was one of the two that matters that triggered his meetings with Dr. Fuentes.

Dr. Navin's main focus in his testimony on this incident was Dr. Fuentes's insistence that he was correct that the patient did not have coronary obstruction. Dr. Navin relied for his view on statements made by surgeons during a morbidity and mortality conference (M&M) that they thought that the patient had a coronary obstruction, based on the heart appearance and on a picture taken during the surgery. Drs. Fuentes and Strong believed that the coronary arteries were not obstructed.

As Dr. Strong, a partner of Dr. Fuentes, testified and as reflected on the sign-out sheet for the patient, the pathology report reflected that there was no cardiac injury and the patient should not have been subjected to surgery. She noted, however, that their cardiology team was outnumbered in the M&M and the surgeons steadfastly held their ground in spite of the pathology report that corroborated Dr. Fuentes's diagnosis and disagreement with Dr. Brauer and her position stated in the M&M. Dr. Navin's critique of Dr. Fuentes for isolating himself from the cardiothoracic surgery service as he advocated his viewpoint on the patient's proper treatment is exactly the type of improper criticism that the AMA, Rosner, and Nanavati all warn against. Indeed, Dr. Navin faulted Dr. Fuentes for advocating his viewpoint.

Nurse Noah's verge is also problematic and not reliable because he stated that a non-physician committed the alleged "workplace [verbal] violence," he destroyed his notes of the event, he wasn't fully paying attention to what was happening between Dr. Fuentes and Dr. Brauer, and there were numerous other witnesses to the alleged confrontation, none of whom were called by the hospital. Dr. Salmon did not observe the interaction between Dr. Fuentes and Dr. Brauer in the patient's room, and when he did meet with them, he testified that Dr. Fuentes acted professionally.

Even though Dr. Fuentes's assessment that there was no coronary obstruction turned out to be correct (as proven by the pathology results), Dr. Brauer performed an operation on the patient, who ultimately died. It is thus especially ironic that Dr. Fuentes is being faulted for endangering a patient when in fact he was advocating for his patient who was unable to advocate for himself and who may have survived without the surgery that was performed on him. Dr. Fuentes's conduct in advocating for his patient in connection with this matter is consistent with the AMA's Code of Ethics and was in no way unjustified.

5. The Non-Patient Safety Interaction

Two years prior, nurse Marc McDonough filed a claim regarding an interaction between Dr. Fuentes and Dr. Samantha Klein, a hospitalist, on the medicine inpatient service. He identified in his complaint the interaction as a "non-patient safety event," thus indicating that it is not proper to consider it under the Nanavati Standard. The claim also reflects that it was to be sent to Mr. Sims and nursing leadership for "follow up," but no close-out for the claim has been produced and it appears that the matter was closed as a non-serious matter.

Moreover, the claim omits the critical fact of Dr. Klein's admission that she yelled at Dr. Fuentes during their interaction, thus undermining the credibility of her assertions in the claim which omit this key point.

Likewise, PA Carmel Asuncion, who witnessed the event, filed a detailed next-day summary and complaint about Dr. Klein's inappropriate conduct during the interaction, which was sent to her supervisor nurse Blevins. Ms. Asuncion detailed also some incredible misconduct by Dr. Brauer in her report, specifically her attempted interference in canceling anesthesia clearance for the patient after Dr. Klein decided to consult her despite Dr. Fuentes. Her report contains several instances of aggressively inappropriate conduct by Dr. Klein, including her admitted yelling in the public hallway at Dr. Fuentes. By contrast, nurse McDonough's verge about the incident omits all of Dr. Klein's inappropriate behavior, rendering it a skewed and misleading rendition of what happened.

While the previous CMO, Dr. Navin, faulted Dr. Fuentes for his interaction with Dr. Klein, perhaps he would have a different view if the hospital had investigated the verge and had he known about Dr. Klein's admitted misconduct, which seems only to have come to light in this hearing.

6. The Final Claim from Cardiothoracic Surgery

Four months prior, a claim was filed against Dr. Fuentes regarding a patient who needed the service of cardiothoracic surgery for aortic repair. The issue that arose was whether the patient could have a minimally invasive procedure by interventional cardiology. Dr. Fuentes consulted with Dr. Marc Reely, the newly appointed mediator, who agreed that the patient should be observed over the weekend before any action was taken. In spite of the agreement brokered by Dr. Reely between Dr. Fuentes and the service, the cardiothoracic surgery service secretly performed a surgical procedure on the patient.

Dr. Reely wrote an email supporting Dr. Fuentes on this issue and testified that he acted according to the agreed-upon protocol. Yet a claim was filed because the cardiothoracic surgery team didn't like the fact that Dr. Fuentes, who the cardiothoracic surgery team had consulted, sought out Dr. Reely's intervention. The cardiothoracic surgery team believed as stated in the verge that this was "going behind our back." However, Dr. Fuentes was exercising his best judgment on behalf of the patient and acting in accordance with protocol and approved by Dr. Reely. It is thus impossible to characterize his conduct as endangering patient care—indeed it seems that unless cardiothoracic surgery gets its way, patients are "considered" endangered by the hospital administration.

7. Hearsay Statements by Nurses and Others

While the Hospital's By-Laws permit the Hearing Officer to consider hearsay evidence, there are strong reasons why he should not, especially when Dr. Fuentes's career is in in the balance and the hearsay at issue is so unreliable.

The long-standing policy disfavoring the admission of hearsay in Anglo–American courts… instructs that [h]earsay is not admissible except as provided by [the evidence] rules or by other law. This general prohibition, subject to various exceptions, reflects that hearsay is presumptively deemed to be untrustworthy and unreliable. The hearsay prohibition ensure[s] the accuracy of the factfinding process by excluding untrustworthy statements, such as those made without the solem-

nity of the oath, and not subject to cross-examination ... or the jury's critical observation of the declarant's demeanor and tone. The risks of admitting hearsay indiscriminately are well known. [S]tatements made out-of-court, not under oath, or not subject to cross-examination may suffer infirmities of perception, memory, and narration if admitted. In addition, there can be an aspect of unfairness, even in civil cases, in the substantive admission of hearsay statements by an absent declarant, without affording the opposing party a chance to cross-examine that person before the fact-finder.[61]

The hospital relies on Mr. Alan Troy interviews and his memorandum summarizing his interviews with nurses and other executives to bolster its claim that Dr. Fuentes "often screams and yells in the cardiology department, creating a hostile work environment." Those anonymous, hearsay statements upon which Mr. Troy relied should not be given any weight. The hospital had the opportunity to subpoena witnesses, and when asked by the Hearing Officer was able to procure the testimony of nurses Simonar, Clark, Noah, and McDonough. At the same time, Dr. Fuentes was also able to secure the testimony of several current hospital employees, all positive. The hospital did not disclose the names of many of the people who Mr. Troy interviewed, and their statements are rank hearsay. Even nurse Clark in his testimony did not corroborate everything that is reflected in Mr. Troy's interview of him and thus it is impossible to know if anything those anonymous individuals said is true.

Moreover, Mr. Troy's statement, based on hearsay, that Dr. Fuentes "does not prioritize patient safety" was directly contradicted by Dr. Grant, the Chief of the Cardiology Department, as well

61 James v Ruiz, 440 NJ Super 45, 59-60, 111 A3d 123, 131-32 [NJ Super Ct App Div 2015](internal citations and quotations omitted).

as by twelve doctors, three nurses, two physicians and four technicians who testified in this case. It would be especially prejudicial to afford weight on this issue that is central to the hospital case.

A prime example of why hearsay should be disregarded is nurse Blevins's complaint. In that complaint he alleged that Dr. Fuentes took "a video of staff while patients are present." Taking a video apparently violates a hospital policy. Had nurse Blevins not been subject to cross-examination, there never would have been his admission that this video-taking assertion was a false allegation. Likewise, had nurse Simonar not been subjected to cross-examination, there never would have been his admission that Dr. Fuentes' colleague apologized to him, contrary to the suggestion in Mr. Troy's notes that Dr. Fuentes had him suppress his complaint about his colleague cursing at him. Finally, during the testimony of Georgina Lark, a cath lab nurse, who was confronted with a claim bearing his name as a victim, did not recall if the event actually happened and denied under oath to have filed any claim against any physician.

8. Racist and Inappropriate Behavior Directed towards Dr. Fuentes

Dr. Fuentes was victimized by a discriminatory animus by both Dr. Brauer and several white nurses who mocked Dr. Fuentes's accent. Technician Miguel de Guerra heard nurse Blevins denigrate Dr. Fuentes publicly, having heard him call him this "F'ing guy" during a meeting. As the court made clear in Nanavati, "allegations of "disharmony" [should] [n]ever be used as a ruse to deny or terminate staff privileges because of a doctor's race, religion, color, or gender."

While nurse Georgina Lark was repeatedly identified as one of the nurses who mocked Dr. Fuentes's accent, she denied doing so. She did concede, however, that she discussed immigration and border crossings at work during the 2020 election cycle and was called to the Human Resources department and warned against discussing politics at work (she also testified that another nurse had the same kind of conversation with human resources).

Notably, although the hospital asked for permission to call nurse Georgina Lark as a rebuttal witness to refute the allegations of discriminatory comments, no request was made by the hospital to recall Dr. Brauer to rebut the allegation made that she mocked Dr. Fuentes's accent in her presence or any of the other nurses who were identified as ones who mocked Dr. Fuentes' accent. Thus, the testimony about Dr. Brauer stands unrebutted. Because the hospital relied so extensively on Dr. Brauer's testimony both in connection with the continuation of the suspension of Dr. Fuentes's privileges and in this hearing, including in connection with the occluded coronary patient and the thoracotomy situation, her discriminatory animus weighs especially heavily.

As detailed previously, Dr. Brauer fabricated a story about Dr. Fuentes causing her to delay performing the thoracotomy. The question then becomes, why did she lie about it? Reeves supports the conclusion that Dr. Brauer lied to cover-up her discriminatory animus. So long as her bias was one of the reasons (her anger about being blamed for the patient's death is another), that's enough to constitute unlawful discrimination.[62] The hospital acted and relied on Dr. Brauer's accusations and as such she was the "cat's paw"

---

62 Bostock v Clayton County, Georgia, 207 L Ed 2d 218, 140 S Ct 1731, 1739 [2020] ("So long as the plaintiff 's sex was one but-for cause of that decision, that is enough to trigger the law.").

for the hospital's actions. Accordingly, unlawful discrimination factored into the hospital adverse decision, which renders it unlawful under the Nanavati Standard.

Beyond Dr. Brauer, the hospital also acted on allegations from the nurses Mr. Troy interviewed, some who harbored racist views of Dr. Fuentes, as evidenced by the mocking of his accent, and thus they were the "cat's paw" that caused the hospital to act. Dr. Fuentes's privileges were thus compromised by an impermissible discriminatory animus in violation of the Nanavati Standard.

9. Dr. Fuentes Treated Staff with Respect and Was a Fierce Patient Advocate

Each of the twenty-two witnesses that Dr. Fuentes called to testify agreed that Dr. Fuentes treated all staff and nurses respectfully, did not yell, and had never done anything to endanger his patients. In fact, most if not all agreed that he was a fierce patient advocate.

10. Dr. Reely's Adverse Testimony Doesn't Satisfy the Nanavati Standard

The hospital called Dr. Marc Reely to support its argument that Dr. Fuentes's view of the correctness of his position in treating patients "probably impacted patient care," supposedly because the cardiothoracic surgery service was dissuaded from offering its views regarding patient care, and that Dr. Fuentes allegedly didn't have insight into how his conduct affected patient care. Notably, Dr. Reely failed to specify any specific examples of any harm to patients to support his generalized claims, rendering his testimony on this point totally useless under the Nanavati Standard, which rejects "general complaints of a physician's inability to cooperate with others" as a basis to revoke privileges.

And, contrary to his allegation elicited on direct examination by the hospital that Dr. Fuentes's conduct was inconsistent with what is required in an HRO, Dr. Reely testified that monthly he referred one or two of his patients to Dr. Fuentes for treatment up until the time he was suspended, which would equal 60-120 patients in total. Dr. Reely admitted that he had no concerns about the safety of those patients because he "trusted Dr. Fuentes to make good decisions with respect to the patients [he] referred to him." The fact that Dr. Reely sent his patients to Dr. Fuentes for treatment undermines and contradicts his testimony that he was a risk to patients. It's a reasonable assumption that Dr. Reely would not have sent patients to Dr. Fuentes for care if there was any potential risk to them.

Moreover, the interview notes taken during Dr. Reely's interview with the four-person investigative subcommittee reflect that Dr. Fuentes has an awareness of when he and other providers disagree: "Demonstrated an awareness as often escalated to CMO for consideration." Thus, his hearing testimony regarding Dr. Fuentes lacking an awareness is directly refuted by his earlier, inconsistent statement to the investigative committee. Indeed, his prior statement reflects that Dr. Fuentes recognized when there was an issue regarding patient care and sought guidance from superior hospital authorities on how to address and resolve those issues.

Further, Dr. Reely was chosen by Dr. Navin as a mediator between Dr. Fuentes and his team, the cardiothoracic surgery service, not just because of Dr. Fuentes, but because of broader issues of disputes that arose regarding the treatment of patients with cardiac issues. Thus, any suggestion that the mediator role was created just for Dr. Fuentes is totally inaccurate.

Dr. Reely was involved in just two or three situations as the mediator (he could only recall two specifically).

In once situation that resulted in a claim being filed by the cardiothoracic surgery service, he agreed that Dr. Fuentes had contacted him to mediate and that he acted in accordance with the agreement that had been reached with the cardiothoracic surgery service, a fact he confirmed in an email to the chairs of surgery and medicine. The cardiothoracic surgery service objected, as noted in the claim, to Dr. Fuentes even involving Dr. Reely as mediator. While the hospital took the cardiothoracic surgery service's side and criticized Dr. Fuentes for invoking Dr. Reely's assistance as the mediator in that situation, he didn't object at the time and in fact helped broker a deal between Dr. Fuentes and the cardiothoracic surgery service for how to treat the patient, a deal that the cardiothoracic surgery proceeded to violate by operating on a patient even though the agreement had been to wait over a weekend to determine if surgery was necessary. Dr. Reely also didn't indicate in his email that Dr. Fuentes had done anything improper in that situation, including soliciting his input as mediator.

The hospital critique of Dr. Fuentes for invoking the mediation process that Dr. Navin had implemented to ensure the best possible outcome for the patient is untethered to any concerns over patient care. Dr. Fuentes was acting within the guidelines of the AMA Code of Ethics in advocating for patient care and under the rules of engagement formulated by Dr. Navin. That is, Dr. Fuentes was operating within the parameters that were established by the hospital as an HRO for addressing a difference of opinion on how to treat patients. He should not be faulted for acting exactly how he was expected to act by his superiors.

The second situation that Dr. Reely recalled where he was mediator was the valve matter involving Dr. Liota. Dr. Reely was initially contacted by Dr. Fuentes and helped mediate between Dr. Fuentes and the cardiothoracic surgery service for the patient to go to the cath lab for the valve adjustment procedure. Dr. Reely did not believe that Dr. Fuentes's care of this patient was improper.

Further, Dr. Fuentes would refer patients to Dr. Reely, and he acknowledged that he did not act in a rigid way when sending him patients for treatment and that he was able to persuade him from time-to-time that his perspective was the better way to treat a patient.

In short, Dr. Reely's testimony that Dr. Fuentes was a risk to patients is based on totally non-specific interactions and thus lacks credibility, and more importantly, lacks legal significance under the Nanavati Standard because of the absence of concrete examples. His testimony also contains exactly the type vague and ambiguous allegations of disharmony that the Rosner case warned against as a basis to revoke privileges.

Moreover, his conclusory statements of harm are refuted by the fact that he sent Dr. Fuentes patients because he trusted his judgement, he was able to persuade him to accept his own medical views, and in the two instances when he was involved as mediator, he acted appropriately. If anything, Dr. Reely's testimony should be read as supporting the view that Dr. Fuentes was a tremendous benefit to the patients admitted to the hospital.

11. The Georgina Lark Mystery Claim

The hospital in its examination of Dr. Fuentes relied on a three-year-old claim where nurse Georgina Lark was supposedly the victim of "workplace violence."

Nurse Georgina Lark, however, denied that she filed the complaint and had no knowledge of what occurred as described in the claim, which was apparently not investigated. This proves that the anonymous computerized claim system is readily abused for improper motives, as Dr. Grant had indicated in the case with nurse Simonar's workplace violence claim, and that uninvestigated allegations aren't trustworthy.

Indeed, in connection with the complaints that were filed against Dr. Fuentes, everyone that was actually investigated (Simonar, Liota, Bauer) was found to lack merit. Nurse Blevins's complaint was also admitted by her to contain a false allegation of video taking/invasion of privacy.

While the hospital criticized Dr. Fuentes for focusing on the outcome of the investigations, he was in fact fully justified in doing so. In each case the individuals who filed the claims had various unrelated motivations.

As the Nanavati Standard makes clear, "unjustified altercations with other doctors or nurses, violations of hospital routines or rules, breaches of professional standards, or the commission of some other act that will adversely affect health care delivery" are what should be considered in revoking hospital privileges. That is, courts assume that there must be merit to an actual concrete complaint before action is taken against a physician.

Thus, it's the merits of each complaint that matter, not the fact that a complaint that was filed. The hospital, by contrast, focused on the existence of the claims and complaints as a basis to criticize Dr. Fuentes, rather than the outcome. Presumably the hospital investigated claims in accordance with HRO principles. Dr. Fuentes should not be punished, as he has been, for focusing on the merits of accusations against him. While the hospital has reason to encourage people to report wrongdoing, as Dr. Grant made clear, false claims should not be used to gain leverage.

> **The lawyer of Dr. Fuentes concluded at the end of the hearing:**
>
> Dr. Fuentes respectfully requests that the Hearing Officer issue a report recommending the rejection of all adverse recommendations by the hospital against Dr. Fuentes and reinstate him retroactively.

Legal Analysis of the Hearing Facts: Top 5 Takeaways

1. The hearing is constructed on behalf of the hospital and against the physician.
2. The burden of proof plays against the physician.
3. There is very limited discovery allowed for the practitioner.
4. Any attempt to justify at all costs the original action(s) taken by the MEC without clear and convincing proofs should not be accepted by the practitioner.
5. Remember that the hospital tribunal can be challenged in state or federal court once you have exhausted all remedies at the hospital level.

CHAPTER 11

THE HEARING OFFICER'S RECOMMENDATION

After a six-month long hearing and its examinations and cross examinations, the hearing officer, at the completion of all interviews, requested a meeting with the different lawyers to discuss the timeline of providing his recommendation and some of the major questions he needed to address.

Here are the questions he was struggling with:

1. What alleged behavior on the part of Dr. Fuentes warranted the precautionary suspension? Which documents and testimony support this suspension?
2. Is Dr. Fuentes, or any physician, not justified in "strongly" supporting his clinical position in order to protect or even save the life of a patient when there exists a disagreement between physicians over the care to be provided? And, how to resolve this question if we only focus on the behavior excluding the clinical scenario at hand?

3. Are there any cases, other than Nanavati v. BTMH, that discuss specific factual scenarios which warrant suspension, termination, or discipline of any kind based upon behavior?
4. How to resolve the seeming contradiction between the testimony from the hospital that Dr. Fuentes could still have had a "full" fair hearing on all issues after an unsuccessful PRC assessment with the email from the hospital lawyer in which it was made clear that Dr. Fuentes needed to waive his hearing rights in order to get the behavior assessment.

Each lawyer submitted their arguments and responded to their best ability to those crucial questions. If this debate would have occurred at the level of a state or federal court, the responses to those questions would have been in Dr. Fuentes's favor. But this was not the case, as Dr. Fuentes was still at the level of the hospital's tribunal.

1. Indeed, even though it was clearly demonstrated that the "perfect storm" event was the event leading to the suspension, the hospital lawyer was really interested in expanding the cause to cover every claim ever made against Dr. Fuentes.
2. When it comes to the ability of physicians to "strongly" defend their patients, according to the hospital, this should happen never! But the AMA position, as well as previous litigation cases (see: chapter 10) have permitted physicians to protect their patients even it means entering into "strong" arguments with other physicians or personnel, as long as they don't break any code of conduct rules or bylaws.
3. Separating the behavior of a physician from the clinical situation at hand is unreasonable, especially when there is a conflict related to a clinical situation—to which concept the hospital vehemently opposed.

4. Concerning the existence of other cases than Nanavati v. BTMH, it was unclear if there were any other legal case covering the topic of physician behavior.
5. Finally, regarding the issue of waiving his hearing right, the hospital lawyer blamed a misunderstanding between both parties, even though the email sent by the hospital lawyer was clearly coercive.

The H.O. demanded an extension of his ten days requirement to present his recommendation and after several delays, attributed to unclear and unrelated reasons, finally delivered his brief two months later.

The Hearing Officer's Recommendation

The Hearing Officer of this process insisted that he allowed both parties to present their respective cases. He saw his task as to assess the initial suspension and its extension by the hospital while considering the burden of proof."

To the biggest surprise of Dr. Fuentes:

1. The H.O. rejected up front that the precautionary suspension, coupled with the requirement to waive his right to a hearing, was de facto a termination.
2. He found that the choice to request a hearing or waive it and adopt the recommendation of the MEC to go to PRC was an acceptable choice.
3. He ruled that the need to select between a hearing or the recommendation of the MEC does not constitute a revocation, nor a coercion.

4. He also insisted that he was asked not to focus on the medical or clinical situation at hand but rather on the behavior.

The H.O. proceeded to analyze the case and objected to Dr, Fuentes's claim of an "inappropriate" initial suspension, since a suspension is designed to prevent danger from occurring while permitting the hospital to further assess the situation. Therefore, expecting accuracy at this early stage is neither required nor reasonable," according to him.

Regarding the initial meeting with Dr. Navin, the H.O. considered it as a clear warning for Dr. Fuentes, and the inability of Dr. Fuentes to see this meeting as such a failure on his part to understand how his behavior was seen by his peers.

The H.O. added that the need to institute a mediator along with the multiple complaints against Dr. Fuentes is further confirmation of Dr. Fuentes' concerning behavior.

The H.O. then assessed claim after claim against Dr. Fuentes and accepted every single one of them as credible while *omitting* that most of them were either rejected by the facts or countered by a witness of Dr. Fuentes during the hearing. He questioned the credibility of Dr. Fuentes when he denied raising his voice or acting unprofessionally in any way.

The H.O. insisted that, irrespective of whether Dr. Fuentes was "correct" regarding his clinical judgment and whatever treatment to offer, his behavior was not productive and could have interfered with the safe delivery of medical care. Most audaciously, he then suggested that all witnesses of Dr. Fuentes either were used to the belligerent manner he communicated with, were loyal to him and saw those who filed those complaints as antagonistic, or likewise felt the same pressures that he did and therefore sympathized with him.

When the H.O. analyzed the "perfect storm" that precipitated the decision to precautionarily suspend Dr. Fuentes, he disagreed with Dr. Grant's assessment of the situation regarding the nurses filing groundless claims to retaliate against Dr. Fuentes, and while admitting that nurse Simonar might have exaggerated Dr. Fuentes's tone, he added that Nurse Clark's testimony alone demonstrated that Dr. Fuentes's behavior was inappropriate and even reconciled their testimonies.

He then referred to the interview of the medical staff president, Dr. Mary Rattner, who cosigned the precautionary suspension that was based on imperfect information and ruled that given the purpose of a precautionary suspension, patient safety supersedes any financial or reputational harm done to a physician by a precautionary suspension.

When addressing the "imperfect investigation" against Dr. Fuentes, the H.O. referred to the Health Care Quality Improvement Act (HCQIA) Act.[63] The HCQIA defines the safe harbor that provides immunity from civil liability regarding the process of corrective action and hearing processes at the level of the hospital and insisted that the HCQIA does not require that the entire investigation related to the action taken meet the specific standard of the law.[64]

Moreover, the HCQIA entitles a practitioner who is the subject of a peer review investigation to a reasonable investigation, *not a perfect investigation.*[65] He also cited the Health Care Act that provides immunity against those involved in peer review functions so long as their actions are in good faith.

---

63 (HCQIA) Act, 42 USC §§11101 et. seq.

64 See, Fobbs v. Holy Cross Health Sys. Corp., 789 F. Supp. 1054 (E. D. Cal. 1992).

65 Egan v. Ethol Mem. Hosp., 102 F. Supp. 798 (S.D. Ohio 1998).

He also ruled that physician behaviors which "may" impact patient care do apply, and there need not be proof of actual patient harm before a hospital is allowed to take action.

The H.O. didn't agree that the leadership of the hospital had any animus against Dr. Fuentes and was convinced that Dr. Fuentes would have been able to come back should he have taken the PRC behavior assessment and wave his hearing right.

He denied that potential racist staff members had any impact (via the cat's paw theory) on Dr. Fuentes's suspension given the other complaints.

When analyzing the thoracotomy incident, while admitting that many witnesses confirmed Dr. Fuentes's version of the event, he noted he could not rely upon this clinical debate to find by clear and convincing evidence that Dr. Fuentes hadn't acted in an inappropriate way, potentially harmful to patients, especially in view of all of the other evidence in the record supporting such a finding.

When confronted with the occluded valve incident, he attributed the whole conflict to an inter-department disagreement and not to Dr. Fuentes's fault. But he accepted Dr. Rattner's recollection of Dr. Fuentes's statement during the Medical Executive Committee Hearing (chapter 4), where allegedly (Dr. Fuentes) blamed everyone but himself and seemed to want to do procedure after procedure with no regard to anything or anybody else. This led the H.O. to conclude that Dr. Rattner's testimony summarized the issues related to Dr. Fuentes's communication style, which were in need for a change.

The H.O. then concluded that Dr. Fuentes did not meet the burden of proof and recommended him to attend an appropriate assessment program to better understand and control his own behavior. This, according to the H.O., may permit the hospital and his patients to benefit from his advanced skills.

When Dr. Fuentes was provided with the hearing officer's decision, which was clearly biased and influenced by the hospital lawyers, he felt like a mouse in a maze without an exit.

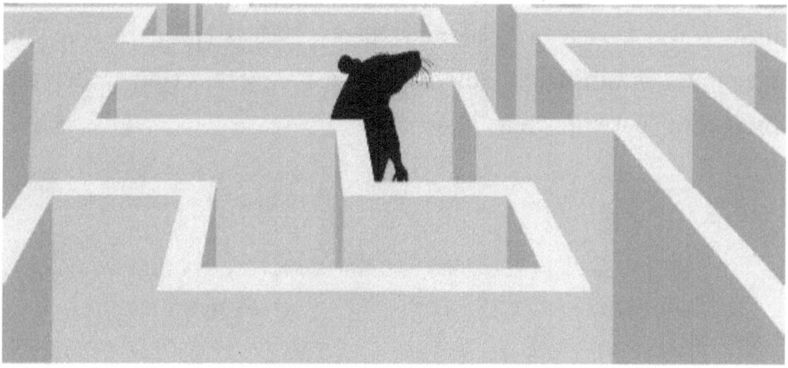

Bias in the H.O.'s Recommendation

Dr. Fuentes's lawyer, Mr. Alan Rogers, was very surprised at how one-sided the hearing officer's conclusion was. The H.O indeed ignored the fact that a year and a half passed, that many due processes were not followed, and that realistically the hospital was not interested in Dr. Fuentes's return. While Dr. Fuentes had no intention to come back to the hospital, he wanted to clear his filing at the NPDB.

Behind the scenes, it was unclear what kind of discussions were happening between the MEC and the legal team of the hospital. Indeed, at that point, the hospital had every reason to resolve this matter as soon as possible, since the whole team of Dr. Fuentes had by then been resigned and moved to a competing institution in Phoenix.

When the legal team of the hospital reached out to Alan Rogers, Dr. Fuentes lawyer, they offered another horrible settlement, with freezing of the current investigation if Dr. Fuentes resigned. This was seen as another attempt to trick Dr. Fuentes, since a resignation at this point would only benefit the hospital and would be reported to the NPDB (see Chapter 5).

What became abundantly clear to Dr. Fuentes and his lawyer was that while the whole suspension, investigation, and hearing process was flawed in so many respects, every step of the way, the hospital was ultimately able to justify its every action under the pretext of "patient safety."

> *The HCQIA of 1986, by granting significant immunity from liability to the peer review processes, including investigative activities and peer review hearings, has permitted hospitals to drag physicians into an endless and unbalanced process aimed at destroying their career if they fail to fall in line.*
>
> *Some states like California have allowed "aggrieved physicians the opportunity to prove that a peer review can be found in court to have been improper due to bad faith or malice, in which case the peer reviewers' immunities from civil liability "fall by the wayside."*[66]

---

66 Greg Abrams, Esq. (May–June 2006). "Attacking Bad Faith Peer Review: Is It a SLAPP?". Sierra Sacramento Valley Medicine. 57 (3). Archived from the original on 2011-07-21.

The Hearing Officer's Recommendation: Top 5 Takeaways

1. Hearing officers are selected and paid by the hospital.
2. Request an independent hearing officer with no previous association with the hospital.
3. The hospital will use the hearing to beef up their case against you.
4. The hearing is not designed to protect the practitioner but rather to create the illusion of a "fair" trial.
5. In most cases, the hearing officer will side with the hospital.

CHAPTER 12

THE APPEAL

Within a month after receipt of the report of the hearing officer, the MEC can affirm, retract, or modify its previous ruling based on the H.O.'s recommendation. If the action of the MEC continues to be against the physician, he or she is then allowed to request an appeal at the level of the hospital board. The physician may request in writing this appeal to the CEO. The written request for an appeal should also include a brief statement of the reasons for appeal.

The CEO of the hospital then has a month to schedule and arrange for the appeal. The CEO then notifies the place, time, and date of the appellate review. The date of the appellate review is typically between one to two months from the date of receipt of the request for appeal.

Grounds for Appeal. The grounds for appeal to the hospital board are typically limited to the following:

a. *There was substantial failure to follow the hospital bylaws so as to deny basic fairness or reasonable due process.*

b. *The recommendation of the hearing officer were made arbitrarily, capriciously, or with prejudice.*

c. *The recommendation of the MEC was not supported by substantial evidence based upon the available record.*

During the appeal process, the board typically considers the record of the hearing before the hearing panel and any written statements submitted by parties to the hearing. Each party typically presents a written statement during the appeal, and all evidence submitted is cross-examined. Additional evidence is accepted if they are new and relevant.

The hospital board or the committee of the board may affirm, modify, or reverse the action that is the subject of the appeal and render a final recommendation. The decision of the board shall be effective immediately and shall not be subject to further review.

At that stage, since the practitioner has fully exhausted the administrative remedies afforded by the bylaws, he or she is then allowed to resort to formal legal action.

A month after receipt of the report of the hearing officer, the MEC decided to affirm its previous recommendation by requesting Dr. Fuentes to attend a behavior assessment program since "his behavior was creating a potential and likely negative impact on patient safety."

The hospital lawyers also had previously reached out to Dr. Fuentes's Lawyer, Mr. Alan Rogers, with an unacceptable settlement for him to resign. Dr. Fuentes decided to appeal to the board of the hospital.

The appeal was based on meeting the requirements delineated above:

a. There was substantial failure to comply prior to the hearing with the provisions contained in the bylaws so as to deny basic fairness or reasonable due process; indeed, the hospital improperly coerced Dr. Fuentes to try and waive his hearing rights; the hospital concealed and destroyed evidence; failed to meet several deadlines clearly delineated in the bylaws; and hired over Dr. Fuentes's timely objection a biased/conflicted hearing officer whose law firm performs services for the hospital.

b. The recommendation of the hearing officer was made arbitrarily, capriciously, and with prejudice; by omitting reference of several key witnesses, rejecting the investigation conducted by Dr. Grant, discrediting improperly every single one of Dr. Fuentes' witnesses, and failing to apply the appropriate standard for his ruling as well as ignoring the clinical situation, which is crucial for any physician interaction in the setting of the hospital.

c. The recommendation of the MEC was not supported by substantial evidence based upon the hearing record; indeed, most witnesses supported that Dr. Fuentes doesn't have any behavior issues nor endangered anyone, and the whole team of Dr. Fuentes resigned in a sign of solidarity, including his partners, nurses, nurse assistants, PA, and XR technicians. Several prominent surgeons from the hospital testified on Dr. Fuentes's behalf that he never endangered any patients or staff and had no behavior issues. Finally, Dr. Fuentes worked for a month without any issue after the inciting incident before being suspended.

The appeal date was set eight weeks later. It is important to note that a year and a half had passed since Dr. Fuentes was first suspended. By that time, the whole team of Dr Fuentes had left the hospital, including his three other interventional cardiologist partners, the two physician assistants, the two advanced instructors, two XR technicians, and dedicated nurses and nurse practitioners. Hence the hospital had no further gain by preventing Dr. Fuentes's rehabilitation and not allowing him to leave after resigning in good standing.

Surviving the Suspension

To deal with the length of the suspension, Dr. Fuentes had to completely adjust his lifestyle:

- He imposed on himself a daily 1-2 hours workout full of cardio to protect his coronaries from stress.
- He had a systematic bimonthly appointment with his therapist to make sure his mental health was in check.
- He worked one to two weeks a month for locum tenens, providing coverage in cardiology.
- He was invited monthly to a national or international conference to lecture on interventional cardiology.
- He was providing consultations including lab experimentation to several industries specialized in cardiologic accessories.
- He connected with his colleagues in Latin America to set up several courses on therapeutic cardiology with live cases, allowing him to keep up with his skillset.
- He took several courses online to improve his communication skills
- He read several books on self enhancement
- He published various review articles in interventional cardiology
- He traveled back to Colombia to visit his parents and childhood friends.

The Appeal Day

On the appeal day, Dr. Fuentes appeared with his lawyer in the auditorium of the hospital. Two weeks prior, both parties had submitted their brief, which were supposedly reviewed by the members of the board. It is important to remember that on the board level, the chairman of medicine, Dr. Friedland doesn't have a seat, while both Dr. Rattner (the medical staff president) and Dr. Livingstone (the CMO) each had a seat, along with Mrs. Laura Browning, the CEO.

A summary of the brief was read by Dr. Rattner on behalf of the CME, summarizing the hearing officer's determination that Dr. Fuentes behavior could eventually endanger staff and/or patients, hence the necessity for him to go an approved behavior assessment. She then discredited Dr. Fuentes for being so poorly collaborative to a process that was meant to bring him back; instead, she insisted Dr. Fuentes made everything so much more difficult by resisting the MEC recommendation and choosing his own behavior assessment.

She failed to mention the need for Dr. Fuentes to waive his hearing right to attend the behavior assessment, all the irregularities of the assessment and processes, as well as the biased hearing officer.

Dr. Fuentes's lawyer was then allowed to make a statement, during which he revisited each ground for appeal as cited above. He focused the majority of his rebuttal on the H.O.'s unfair ruling that ignored some key witnesses and discredited all other witnesses supporting Dr. Fuentes. The H.O. also didn't trust Dr. Grant's investigation, nor did he find Dr. Fuentes having to wave his hearing right irregular.

Finally, the board decided to hear from Dr. Fuentes. He decided to show a humble demeanor hoping to convince the board to reinstate him. He stated that his communication style due to culture or linguistic difference might have been a component of the matter with the hospital. He recognized that he was a very assertive and confident person, and this might be intimidating for some staff, as he was a strong patient advocate.

He also said that while there was no proof of any patient harm, he nevertheless took it upon himself to go to the assessment performed by Vanderbilt in Nashville, since the PCR assessment was unavailable to meet the MEC's recommendation.

Dr. Fuentes also pointed out that the matter with the hospital is much more complex since his whole team resigned, moreover many of those nurses accusing Dr. Fuentes have now participated in a long strike against the hospital and eventually resigned. He also insisted that while looking into the behavior assessments, Dr. Fuentes was made aware of several career-ending stories related to those behavior assessment programs. Indeed, those behavior assessment programs have a growing reputation for not being fully accredited and not using forensic psychiatrists.

After his statement, Dr. Fuentes was excused and the board meeting was adjourned for two weeks to reconvene for a final decision.

The Final Decision of the Hospital Board

The final decision of the hospital board came by certified mail. The board had decided to sustain the decision of the MEC and gave Dr. Fuentes a month to obey to the recommendation by enrolling in the only behavior assessment program they offered from the beginning, the PRC. It again emphasized that his failure to do so will result with termination of his privileges.

The letter also insisted that, according to the hospital bylaws, any type of mental, behavioral, and/or physical assessment can required by the President, CEO, CMO, and/or MEC when it appears necessary to protect the well-being of patients and/or staff and as part of an evaluation of the member's ability to exercise his privileges safely and efficiently.

The letter ended with the statement that Dr. Fuentes had exhausted all remedies at the hospital level.

After a year and half of battling at the hospital level in a biased and unfair system where a claim of potential danger was totally manufactured and a behavior assessment was only used to delay and ruin Dr. Fuentes's reputation, he was finally able to pursue his litigation in court.

The Appeal: Top 5 Takeaways

1. The hospital board has ultimate authority over legal and regulatory processes.
2. The appeal at the board level is the last step before before taking your case to a state or federal court.
3. In most cases the board of the hospital will enforce the recommendation of the Medical Executive committee.
4. The statement of your case presented to the board will constitute, in most cases, the grounds for the lawsuit.
5. Any settlement opportunity before going to court can be attempted at this stage of the process.

CHAPTER 13

THE LAWSUITS

Mr. Alan Rogers, Dr. Fuentes's lawyer, had no other option than to file an appeal of the H.O. decision at the federal or state level to prevent the hospital from revoking Dr. Fuentes's privileges.

Already, Dr. Fuentes had filed a discrimination lawsuit at the federal level and a defamation lawsuit at the state level against the nurses and some of the physicians that testified against him during the hearing.

It is important to recognize that the appeal of the board's decision in court has to identify flaws in the H.O. decision. That's why the appeal at the hospital level set the stage for the appeal in court. Alan Rogers knew that the strongest point of the appeal is the conflicting ruling of the H.O. where in another, earlier case he used the Nanavati for a suspended physician while later he said it didn't apply to Dr. Fuentes's case because he was suspended and not terminated.

Within a week, Dr. Fuentes's lawyer filed the appeal case in the state of Arizona and requested a mediation meeting with the judge assigned to the case.

Importantly, the state of Arizona was suffering from a major shortage of judges, many of them retiring during the Covid-19 pandemic, hence a mediation meeting with an attempt at settlement is always preferred at the civil level.

A month later, a mediation meeting was set up in the personal office of state Judge Patrick Harrison. The terms of the settlement offered by Dr. Fuentes were as follows. *In order for Dr. Fuentes to release the hospital from all litigations against all its personal, he requested:*

1. The filling at the NPDB to be voided, since no specific patient issue was raised.
2. Acceptance of the Nashville course as an approved assessment.
3. Reinstatement of privileges (with resignation as soon as reinstated).
4. Removal of the one year non-compete clause within 10 miles in the state of Arizona.

Unfortunately, the administration of the hospital via the hospital lawyer had no desire to void the NPBD filing, arguing that the hospital would be liable for not reporting the behavior of Dr. Fuentes and declined to waive the non-compete under the specific order of the CEO fearing that Dr. Fuentes would become a major competitor.

NPDB Filling and Sanction for the Hospital

A "Void Report "is processed when the hospital determines that the report was filed in error, did not comply with NPDB reporting guidelines, or an authorized committee has voted to vacate the initial adverse action (e.g., summary suspension). All of these reasons for voiding a damaging report that a hospital has filed with the data bank would place the hospital in a position of significant liability.

Hospitals often justify the refusal of voiding the NPDB filing by referencing the regulation below:

> *HCQIA 42 U.S.C. §11111(b): If the Secretary of the department of Health and Human Services (HHS) believes that a hospital failed to report information in accordance with section 11133 (a) of this title, the Secretary can investigate the hospital. If, after providing notice of noncompliance, an opportunity to correct the noncompliance, and an opportunity for a hearing, the Secretary determines that a health care entity has failed substantially to report information in accordance with section 11133 (a) of this title, the Secretary will publish the name of the entity in the Federal Register. The protections of subsection (a)(1) of this section shall not apply to a hospital, the name of which is published in the Federal with respect to professional review actions for a 3-year period beginning 30 days after the date of publication.*
>
> *Interestingly, the Secretary does not engage in random visits to hospitals to see if they are properly reporting Adverse Actions or not. The question then arises, who would report a hospital's failure to report an Adverse Action to the NPDB? The*

> *hospital itself? The physician against whom the hospital implemented an Adverse Action? There is no evidence that the Secretary has ever imposed the penalty specified in §11111(b). There is also no evidence that the Secretary has ever taken any action against a hospital for failing to report an Adverse Action*
>
> *Finally, §11111(b) provides a hospital with the opportunity to "correct the noncompliance" and an opportunity for a hearing. Thus, hospitals are treated quite fairly regarding NPBD reporting. A hospital would be provided with an opportunity to correct the noncompliance of a reportable action in the unlikely event that someone complains to the secretary that the hospital has not complied.*[67]

Dr. Fuentes's three lawsuits proceeded simultaneously.

1. The state level appeal of the Hearing Officer's decision
2. The federal level discrimination lawsuit
3. The state level defamation lawsuit

Preliminary Injunction (PI)

After filling the appeal of the hearing officer's decision at the state level, Dr. Fuentes's lawyer filed a preliminary injunction to reinstate Dr. Fuentes's privileges pending the final decision of the court regarding the appeal.

67 ref: Sham Summary Suspension: Injunctions to Prevent Irreparable HarmJournal of American Physicians and Surgeons Volume 26 Number 3 Fall 2021

The purpose of a PI is to maintain the status quo pending completion of litigation.[68] The status quo generally consists of the last actual, peaceable, lawful, and non-contested status that predated litigation.[69]

The U.S. Supreme Court, in the case of Winter v. Natural Resources Defense Council, Inc., established a universal standard in federal court for a PI.[70] But the way courts have interpreted and applied these standards varies.[71]

The "Winter Factors" can be summarized below.

- The court must determine that the plaintiff is likely to succeed on the merits.
- The court must determine that the plaintiff is likely to suffer irreparable harm if the injunction is not granted.
- The court must determine that the balance of harms/equities favors the plaintiff—that is, the plaintiff will suffer greater harm if the injunction is not granted than the harm suffered by the defendant(s) if the injunction is granted.
- The court must determine that granting the injunction will not disserve the public interest.

Unfortunately for Dr. Fuentes, the judge decided to reject the pre-

---

68 Cornell Law School. Preliminary injunction. Legal Information Institute. Available at: https://www.law.cornell.edu/wex/preliminary_injunction.Accessed Aug 12, 2021.\

69 Pa. PUC v. Israel, 356 Pa. 400, 406, 52A.2d 317, 321 (1947).

70 Winter v. Natural Resources Defense Council, Inc. 555 U.S. 7 (2008). Available at: https://supreme.justia.com/cases/federal/us/555/7/. Accessed Aug 12, 2021.

71 Moore MD. The preliminary injunction standard: understanding the publicinterest factor. Michigan Law Review 2019;117(5):938-961. Available at: https://repository.law.umich.edu/cgi/viewcontent.cgi?article=2513&context=mlr.Accessed Aug 12, 2021.

liminary injunction based on the facts that the irreparable harm has already happened (i.e., the NPDB filling and inability to secure a new position), and it was not clear that the plaintiff would suffer greater harm if the injunction was not granted.

At that stage, the appeal of the hearing officer decision had to follow its course in court.

The Appeal of the Hearing Officer's Decision at the State Level

The Hearing Officer expressly rejected in his decision the legal argument advanced by Dr. Fuentes's lawyer, which was that his conduct needed to be evaluated under the standard developed by the "Nanavati Standard."[72] Specifically, under the Nanavati Standard, he argued that the hospital was required to establish that "prospective disharmony [between himself and others] will ***probably have an adverse impact on patient care.***" (emphasis added) but, this was not the articulated basis for Dr. Fuentes's continued suspension. Rather the hospital decided that "your behavior towards other healthcare professionals created a potential and likely negative impact on patient safety." This was a legal error and constitutes cause for reversal under the hospital by-laws that this action was "arbitrary, capricious or with prejudice."

Appellate courts have at least twice addressed a physician's suspension or disciplinary actions as less severe than revocation of privileges and have in both instances applied the Nanavati Stan-

---

72 Nanavati v Burdette Tomlin Mem. Hosp., 107 NJ 240, 254, 526 A2d 697, 704 [1987]

dard in evaluating the case. In Courtney v Shore Memorial Hospital, the state court heard an appeal from a physician challenging a one-year penalty of supervised probation for "disruptive behavior" stemming from dozens of different complaints against him. The court in *Courtney* explained that,

> *Nanavati* deals with disharmony—personality difficulties which are largely subjective and in a reasonably large institution inevitable. *Id.* at 253, 526 *A.*2d 697. It is only when conduct reaches the level of interfering with patient care that it can be penalized. *Id.* at 253–255, 526 *A.*2d 697. Thus, the standard requires the hospital to establish that "prospective disharmony will probably have an adverse impact on patient care." *Id.* at 254, 526 *A.*2d 697. "Prospective" because the sanction is intended to protect patient care, not punish a doctor for past personality failures.245 NJ Super. at 142.[73]

In Courtney, the hospital board made a finding expressly under the Nanavati Standard and the Court held that, "Suffice it to say that we are satisfied that the Board's findings were supported by sufficient reliable evidence and that the hospital established that prospective disharmony will probably have an adverse impact on patient care, essentially for the reasons given by the trial judge in his oral opinion of October 19, 1989."

There was no dispute that the Nanavati Standard applied in Courtney to a "supervised probation," which is clearly less severe

---

73 Courtney v Shore Mem. Hosp., 245 NJ Super 138, 139, 584 A2d 817, 818 [NJ Super Ct App Div 1990], t

than a revocation of privileges. Like the physician in Courtney, Dr. Fuentes's conduct should have been evaluated under the Nanavati Standard. It was not, and instead it was evaluated under a less exacting standard to his prejudice.

In *Ramamurthy v JFK Medical Center*, the Court addressed a physician's 90-day suspension due to his conduct, which led to a patient's death. The court explained,

> Where a court reviews a decision of a hospital board, it "should focus on the reasonableness of the action taken" with reference to the "interests of the public, the applicant and the hospital." *Garrow v. Elizabeth Gen. Hosp. & Dispensary*, 79 *N.J.* 549, 565 (1979). The standard of review of a hospital board's determination is less rigorous than the substantial credible evidence test, as "the record should contain sufficient reliable evidence, even though of a hearsay nature, to justify the result." *Ibid. See Nanavati v. Burdette Tomlin Mem'l Hosp.*, 107 *N.J.* 240, 249 (1987). Practitioners subject to corrective action are entitled to fundamental fairness, which requires notice of the charges against them as well as a hearing. *Garrow, supra,* 79 *N.J.* at 558 (citing *Cunningham v. Dep't of Civil Serv.*, 69 *N.J.* 13, 19 (1975)). Fundamental fairness provides a limited right to counsel as well as limited pre-hearing disclosure of the hospital's basis for bringing the corrective action. *Zoneraich v. Overlook Hosp.*, 212 *N.J.Super.* 83, 91 (App.Div.), *certif. denied*, 107 *N.J.* 32 (1986).[74]

74 Ramamurthy v JFK Med. Ctr., A-4579-08T1, 2010 WL 2010993, at *1 [NJ Super Ct App Div May 21, 2010],

Although the Court in *Ramamurthy* did not directly address the issue of whether the physician's conduct would "probably have an adverse impact on patient care," as required under the Nanavati Standard, nonetheless the court's citation to the *Nanavati* case lends strong support for the conclusion that the Nanavati Standard applies to suspensions and other actions less severe than revocation of privileges.

Indeed, a failure to adhere precisely to the strict standard delineated under the Nanavati Standard has been found to deprive a physician of a fair hearing as a matter of law, requiring the reversal of a hospital board's decision revoking a physician's privileges. "Application of a less exacting standard for his conduct to impact patient care prejudiced [the physician's] right to a fair hearing."[75]

It is telling that the Hearing Officer argued so vigorously against the application of the Nanavati Standard to Dr. Fuentes' case, obviously recognizing that the allegations asserted against him would not warrant any adverse action under the Nanavati Standard.

Further, rather than determining that the Nanavati Standard applied, and instead of using any standard drawn from the By-Laws, or from any court decision, or even any standard articulated by the Hearing Officer in his Decision, the Hospital formulated its own *ad-hoc* standard to justify Dr. Fuentes continued suspension. That standard, "your behavior towards other healthcare professionals created a potential and likely negative impact on patient safety" was newly minted for Dr. Fuentes and was based on no authoritative source.

---

75 anavati v Cape Regional Med. Ctr., A-4111-17T3, 2020 WL 2529523, at *5 [NJ Super Ct App Div May 19, 2020].

Interestingly, the reason for his continued precautionary suspension was based on "the reasonable possibility that the failure to do so may pose danger to the health or safety of any individual or the orderly operation of the Hospital." This statement was based on (a) false and defamatory claims that nurse Simonar filed alleging "workplace violence," the view that Dr. Fuentes focuses on the favorable outcome for him of variety of "incidents" as opposed to focusing on an alleged broader theme that supposedly triggers the "incidents," and (c) "challenges related to interpersonal communications" between certain doctors and Dr. Fuentes that supposedly "jeopardize [those doctors'] ability to care for patients to the best of their ability and influence willingness to request future consultations from Dr. Fuentes.

Taken together, the hospital has formulated differing and shifting grounds for the suspension, none of which find any support in the by-laws or in the state law.

Judge Patrick Harrison's Acceptance of the Case

After reviewing the legal argument provided to challenge the hearing officer's ruling, State Judge Patrick Harrison agreed that the Nanavati Standard should have been used to assess Dr. Fuentes's conduct. He then ruled that the hearing at the hospital didn't apply the appropriate standard, hence Dr. Fuentes needed to be offered a new hearing in civil court.

This took the hospital legal team by surprise, objecting that the hearing should be redone at the hospital, but the judge was very concerned with the timeline, indeed more than a year and half has passed since Dr. Fuentes was initially suspended, and Dr. Fuentes's lawyer had raised many concerns in his appeal to the Judge.

The Hearing Officer's decision overlooked or misconstrued critical evidence, compelling the conclusion that the decision was not supported by substantial evidence based on the hearing record, in violation of the by-laws. The proof of this conclusion includes the fact that:

- **The H.O. accepted the statement of Dr. Rattner to suspending Dr. Fuentes one month after the peak event** since he supposedly "interfered" with a code (he did not, as confirmed by the video footage and all the testimonies) and in the afternoon engaged in loud yelling with the nurses to bring unsafely an intubated patient down (the sign out and several testimonies demonstrated that the intubated patient was never brought down and Nurse Clark herself acknowledged twice that Dr. Fuentes didn't yell.
- **The H.O. completely ignored critical testimony from Dr. Reely**, appointed as a mediator between the cardiology department and the cardiothoracic surgery team, that Dr. Fuentes always acted properly under the mediation system instituted and that he trusted Dr. Fuentes so much that he regularly sent him patients until his suspension. The decision's failure to address his testimony is significant, because he was the hospital witness and the omission can only be seen as willful ignorance of evidence that does not fit into the narrative that the hospital wanted to advance, which was that Dr. Fuentes is a danger to patients. The decision's failure to address Dr. Reely's testimony also supports the conclusion that the decision is arbitrary and capricious, with the Hearing Officer cherry-picking the evidence to exclude compelling exculpatory evidence.

- **The H.O.'s decision omits any reference to the testimony of Dr. Natacha Romanov.** The hospital accused Dr. Fuentes of disruptive behavior in his interactions with Dr. Janet Brauer, but the Hearing Officer failed to address Dr. Romamov's testimony, ignoring exculpatory testimony, further bolstering the conclusion that his decision was crafted to support the hospital's favored outcome and that any evidence that would undermine that conclusion would be ignored. He offered no reason why Dr. Romanov wasn't credible. He simply ignored evidence that didn't fit the hospital's preferred narrative.
- **The H.O. found credible that a nurse had filed an anonymous complaint** against Dr. Fuentes when in fact the nurse expressly denied under oath that she had anything to do with the claim and had no knowledge of the facts and circumstances recounted in the claim. It was arbitrary and capricious for the Hearing Officer to credit the validity of this anonymous verge when its alleged author (or the victim of the events described in it) testified that he had no connection to or knowledge of any facts relating to it.
- **The H.O. rejected the testimony of nurse Clark**, who claimed multiple times that Dr. Fuentes did not yell at her, a conclusion that Dr. Grant also reached after investigating and rejecting nurse Simonar's complaint that Dr. Fuentes yelled at nurse Clark aggressively. Dr. Grant concluded in his report on nurse Simonar's verge that he "us[ed] threats to harm the reputations of the physicians, such as claiming violence, when in this case there was none" in order to gain leverage in working out differences. The Hearing Officer offered no reason to disregard Dr. Grant's conclusions about this claim (it was the so-called "perfect storm" event that triggered Dr. Fuentes' precautionary suspension), when he gave deference

to and credited Dr. Grant's other investigation (i.e., rejecting Dr. Liota's claim). Indeed, the Hearing Officer clearly ignored the substantial evidence that Dr. Fuentes did not yell at nurse Clark, because to credit that story would undermine the entire premise on which the precautionary suspension was first implemented and would thus rip away the foundation of the hospital case against him.

- **The H.O. found none of the witnesses of Dr. Fuentes credible, stating** "that these individuals had become used to Dr. Fuentes' fashion of communication or that they too felt the same pressures that he did to get as many cases done as possible and therefore commiserated with him. It may also be that they felt a sense of loyalty to him or that they saw those who had filed verges and complaints as 'the problem.'" This statement is not only erroneous since those witnesses not only included other cardiologists, but also nurses, nurses' assistants, and radiation technicians who would not benefit from "doing more cases" but also two senior surgeons and a senior anesthesiologist (Dr. Romeo Sabatini) who have no sense of loyalty towards him and still work at the hospital.
- **The H.O., when assessing the thoracotomy event**, could not find by clear and convincing evidence that Dr. Fuentes didn't act in an inappropriate and potentially harmful way to patients, **totally ignoring five witnesses**.

The Federal Lawsuits

In the case of Dr. Fuentes, the federal lawsuits included three options:

1. The Antitrust Lawsuit
2. The Fraud Lawsuit
3. The Discrimination Lawsuit

The Antitrust Lawsuit[76]

A hospital may be found in violation of antitrust laws if it takes action against a physician's medical staff membership for anti-competitive reasons.[77] For instance, the hospital uses its peer reviewed process as a means of eliminating competition. Such action may violate the Sherman Act and/or state antitrust laws.[78] Violations of these laws can entail costly litigation, treble damages, and civil or criminal penalties.[79]

---

76 Sham Peer Review: Antitrust Concerns Journal of American Physicians and Surgeons Volume 28 Number 2 Summer 2023

77 15 U.S.C. §§ 1, 2 (2021). Section 1 states that "[every] contract . . . or conspiracy, in restraint of trade or commerce . . . is hereby declared to be illegal." Section 2 states: "Every person who shall monopolize, or attempt to monopolize, or combine or conspire with any other person or persons, to monopolize any part of the trade or commerce . . . shall be deemed guilty of a felony"; see also 15 U.S.C. § 45 (1988) (deeming unfair methods of competition unlawful).

78 E.g., Alaska. Stat. § 45.50.564 (2021); Del. Code. Ann., tit. 6 §§ 2101-14 (2022); Mich. Comp. Laws §§ 445.771–.788 (2021).

79 15 U.S.C. § 15(a). Additionally, because violation of the Sherman Act is considered a felony, it is grounds for mandatory exclusion from participation in Medicare and state health care programs—a death knell for most providers. 42 U.S. C. § 1320a-7(a)(1).

To establish a claim under Section 1 of the Sherman Act, a plaintiff must establish four elements:

1. a contract, combination, or a conspiracy,[80]
2. a substantial impact on interstate commerce,
3. an anti-competitive purpose or effect, and
4. an effect on relevant services and markets.[81]

However, physicians have rarely been successful in bringing antitrust claims, largely because of the difficulty of proving antitrust violations in this context.[82] Specifically, the antitrust laws were designed to protect competition, as opposed to competitors, and, as noted by the Fourth Circuit, "The fact that a hospital's decision caused a disappointed physician to practice medicine elsewhere does not of itself constitute an antitrust injury."[83] Furthermore, hospitals have a defense against antitrust claims if they can show that they acted for a reason independent of any anti-competitive motivations, such as quality of care.[84] They will use the immunity provided under the HCQIA.

---

80 Legal authority is divided on whether the medical staff is a separate legal entity for purposes of conspiring with the hospital. E.g., Wallace v. Garden City Hosp. Osteopathic, 330 N.W.2d 850 (Mich. 1983); cf. Oltz v. St. Peter's Cmty. Hosp., 861 F.2d 1440 (9th Cir. 1988); Weiss v. York Hosp., 745 F.2d 786 (3d Cir. 1984); Bolt v. Halifax Hosp. Med. Ctr., 851 F.2d 1273 (11th Cir. 1988).

81 e.g., Bus. Elecs. Corp. v. Sharp Elecs. Corp., 485 U.S. 717 (1988).

82 E.g., Novak v. Somerset Hosp., 625 F. App'x 65 (3d Cir. 2015); Patel v. Midland Mem'l Hosp. & Med. Ctr., 298 F.3d 333 (5th Cir. 2002); BCB Anesthesia Care v. Passavant Mem'l Area Hosp. Ass'n, 36 F. 3d 664 (7th Cir. 1994); Austin v. McNamara, 979 F.2d 728 (9th Cir. 1992).

83 Brown Shoe Co. v. United States, 370 U.S. 294 (1962); see also Oksanen v. Page Mem'l Hosp., 945 F.2d 696 (4th Cir. 1991) (en banc); Todorov v. DCH Healthcare Auth., 921 F.2d 1438 (11th Cir. 1991).

84 E.g., Matthews v. Lancaster Gen. Hosp., 87 F.3d 624 (3d Cir. 1996); Robinson v. Magovun, 688 F.2d 824 (3d Cir. 1982).

Indeed, the HCQIA provides that a professional review body (of a hospital) shall not be liable for damages where the actions are taken:

1. in the reasonable belief that the action was in the furtherance of quality health care
2. after a reasonable effort to obtain the facts of the matter
3. after adequate notice and hearing procedures are afforded to the physician involved or after such procedures as are fair to the physician under the circumstances
4. in the reasonable belief that the action was warranted by the facts known after such reasonable effort to obtain facts and after meeting the requirements of paragraph (3).[85]

The Fraud Lawsuit

Dr. Fuentes also had grounds for a fraud lawsuit. The components of his fraud lawsuit are as follows:

1. *A Notice letter was sent by hospital administration claiming that the hearing would be conducted according to the medical staff bylaws. The bylaws were attached to the notice letter. However, the hospital leaders did not follow the medical staff bylaws, as evidenced by the fact they repeatedly violated them so as to achieve the desired outcome during the process. Dr. Fuentes reasonably relied on this misrepresentation and was harmed as a result.*[86]
2. *The attorney representing the hospital and a member of the investigation committee falsely implicated Dr. Fuentes in interfering*

85 Health Care Quality Improvement Act (HCQIA), 42 U.S.C. §§ 11101–11151.

86 Sham Peer Review: the Ultimate Fraud Journal of American Physicians and Surgeons Volume 28 Number 4 Winter 2023

with a thoracotomy, based on the false allegation that during the procedure he delayed the surgeon to perform the thoracotomy. Dr. Fuentes was harmed as a result of this misrepresentation.

3. *The attorney representing the hospital and medical staff president held meetings at which they discussed how they were going to delay the return of Dr. Fuentes as to achieve the desired outcome—removing the physician from the hospital and ruining his medical career. Part of the plan was to use false charges of interfering with a code on the morning of the spike event and bringing in an unsafe manner an intubated patient to the coronary care unit in the afternoon of the same day. The hospital attorney, medical staff president, and HR director, in order to create a file against Dr. Fuentes, then conspired to knowingly file a false databank report against Dr. Fuentes. Dr. Fuentes was harmed as a result of this conspiracy.*

The Discrimination Lawsuit

Third, the claims behind a discrimination lawsuit include:

1. *The hospital suspended Dr. Fuentes's privileges based on false allegations that he had engaged in "workplace violence." Those "workplace violence" charges were filed by a disgruntled and poorly performing nurse, who had made plans prior to filing his complaint to leave the hospital for a nursing job in a nursing home. His allegations of "workplace violence" were thoroughly investigated and rejected by the chief of cardiology. Nonetheless, after his initial suspension on, the HR began a selective process to seek statements from nurses and others to use against Dr. Fuentes. Nurses and others in the department who were favorable to Dr. Fuentes weren't interviewed. Several anonymous statements were*

taken and used by the hospital to continue his suspension. The HR department omitted exculpatory statements that were favorable to Dr. Fuentes in a memorandum presented to the medical staff.

2. *The HR director made an inflammatory and defamatory presentation in Dr. Fuentes's presence to the medical staff, in an effort to secure his suspension, based on what the selective group of nurses and others had said in their interviews, and she shredded his notes of that presentation and took actions to ensure that there was no record of his notes, including failing to save them on his computer.*
3. *Among the nurses who provided statements against Dr. Fuentes, several nurses openly ridiculed the accent of Dr. Fuentes (born in Colombia from Latin American parents), which is a heavy Hispanic accent. This same group of nurses made discriminatory anti-Hispanic comments to several staff technicians and doctors.*
4. *Another hospital-employed physician, Dr. Janet Brauer, was also overheard to have ridiculed Dr. Fuentes's accent. Some of the staff who had been targeted for anti-Hispanic and racist comments by the nurses in question complained to the HR department, but their complaints were ignored. Dr. Fuentes did not learn about the discriminatory comments until the "Fair Hearing," when sworn testimony was provided establishing that these comments were made.*

The working hypothesis is the hospital, in seeking to keep labor peace with the nurses due to the severe nursing shortage in Arizona, acted on the nurses' complaints and orchestrated Dr. Fuentes's suspension. Several nurses who complained about Dr. Fuentes harbored a discriminatory animus towards him based on his national origin and/or ethnic Hispanic ancestry, as evidenced through their ridiculing of his accent. The hospital acted under a cat's paw theory to suspend Dr. Fuentes and seek the removal of his privileges based on nurses who harbored a discriminatory animus and who also created a hostile environment in the cath lab.

Dr. Janet Brauer similarly harbored a discriminatory animus towards Dr. Fuentes based on ridiculing his accent and her comments made to the medical staff during its investigation, which were tinged with a discriminatory animus. Dr. Rattner was also personally involved in helping orchestrate Dr. Fuentes's suspension, when she directed a scheme that Dr. Fuentes take an assessment course offered by a third-party.

Dr. Fuentes's suspension has been very costly to his professional reputation as one of the world's leading interventional cardiologists. His suspension has allowed rumors that he acted in inappropriate ways to circulate without correction. He lost his substantial medical practice, and has been unable to attend to patients. He also incurred substantial legal fees in challenging his suspension. He believes that at least one or more of the factors that resulted in his suspension is his national origin and/or Hispanic ancestry.

The process for filing a discrimination lawsuit involves filing an official claim in writing to the ***US Equal Employment Opportunity Commission (EEOC).*** *When a charge is filed against an organization, the EEOC will review the claim and respond with two possibilities:*

1. *The EEOC can reject the claim upfront*
2. *The EEOC can accept the claim and request a response from the hospital.*

During the investigation, the hospital and the physician will be asked to provide information. The EEOC investigator will evaluate the information submitted and make a recommendation as to whether there is reasonable cause to believe that unlawful discrimination has taken place. The hospital may be asked to:

- *submit a statement of position. This is the institution's opportunity to tell its side of the story.*
- *respond to a Request for Information (RFI). The RFI may ask the institution to submit personnel policies, the charging party's personnel files, the personnel files of other individuals, and other relevant information.*
- *permit an on-site visit. Such visits greatly expedite the fact-finding process and may help achieve quicker resolutions. In some cases, an on-site visit may be an alternative to an RFI if requested documents are made available for viewing or photocopying.*
- *provide contact information for or have employees available for* ***witness interviews****. A representative of the hospital may be present during interviews with management personnel, but the EEOC investigator is allowed to conduct interviews of non-management level employees without the presence or permission of the institution.*

Once the investigator has completed the investigation, EEOC will make a determination on the merits of the charge.

- *If the EEOC is unable to conclude that there is reasonable cause to believe that discrimination occurred, the charging party will be issued a notice called a* ***Dismissal and Notice of Rights.*** *This notice informs the physician that s/he has the right to file a lawsuit in federal court within 90 days from the date of its receipt. The hospital will also receive a copy of this notice.*
- *If the EEOC determines there is reasonable cause to believe discrimination has occurred, both parties will be issued a* ***Letter of Determination*** *stating that there is reason to believe that discrimination occurred and inviting the parties to join the agency in seeking to resolve the charge through an informal process known as* ***conciliation****.*

➔ *When conciliation does not succeed in resolving the charge, the EEOC has the authority to enforce violations of its statutes by filing a lawsuit in federal court. If the EEOC decides not to litigate, the physician will receive a* ***Notice of Right to Sue*** *and may file a lawsuit in federal court within 90 days.*

The Lawsuits: Top 5 Takeaways

1. The most common pathway in court is a state-level appeal of the board or Hearing Officer's decision.
2. It is very difficult to bring an antitrust claim, since the hospital will use the immunity provided under the HCQIA.
3. It is also challenging to bring a discrimination lawsuit against the hospital, since it requires a direct relation between the discrimination and the hospital's action.
4. A fraud lawsuit requires the demonstration of communications aiming at creating a false narrative in order to sanction a physician.
5. By the time the practitioner arrives in court, the hospital has created a large file to defend its actions.

CHAPTER 14

THE FINAL OUTCOME

After weighing all the options, Mr. Alan Rogers, Dr. Fuentes's lawyer, recommended to focus on the defamation lawsuit to be filed as a civil state lawsuit. Indeed, the antitrust and fraud lawsuit would be very difficult to win since the hospital, protected by the health care act, will use every incident and the file created against Dr. Fuentes to try to win the case.

The Discrimination Lawsuit Outcome

The hospital responded to the allegation of discrimination made by Dr. Fuentes by pointing out:

1. That Nanavati v. Burdette Tomlin Memorial Hosp., 107 NJ 240, 526 A.2d 697 (1987), heavily cited by Mr. Alan Rogers, was ultimately rejected by the hearing officer. Moreover, the physician whose privileges were revoked in the Nanavati litigation also sued the hospital in federal court for, among other things, breach of Title VII on the grounds that the hos-

pital had revoked his privileges due to his race and national origin. The federal district court dismissed the Title VII cause of action because the physician was not an employee covered by Title VII. Nanavati v. Burdette Tomlin Memorial Hosp., 1986 WL 15318 at *3 (D.N.J. June 23, 1986) ("In the performance of his work at the Hospital—the diagnosis and treatment of patients—Dr. Nanavati makes his own independent decisions regarding patient care, carring [sic] out his activities in the manner he believes to be best for his patients. The Hospital does not have the right to control the 'means and manner' of his work performance. In addition, the practice of medicine, a highly specialized and skilled profession, is generally practiced without extensive supervision.") (appended as Exhibit 9). The physician conceded that determination by not appealing it. Nanavati v. Burdette Tomlin Memorial Hosp., 857 F.2d 96, 111 (3d Cir.1988) ("Nanavati has not appealed the district court's dismissal of the Title VII claim").

2. Dr. Fuentes's national origins are not readily ascertainable, and the hospital has no record of where he was born or the race to which he identifies.
3. His national origin & race are not easily apparent.
4. The Complaints Were Not Animated by Dr. Fuentes's National Origin or Race but rather by "his behavior."
5. Dr. Fuentes never Claim that the Hospital decided to conduct its investigation because of his National Origin or Race.
6. The Hospital Imposed the Suspension Only After Due Deliberation, and it Has Been Independently Investigated and Assessed Multiple Times – With Identical Results.
7. The Cat's Paw Theory of Liability Has No Application and detailed. The Hospital's decision-making process and deci-

sion making was not infected. None of the complainants acted with a discriminatory motive; their accusations were not false; the Hospital did not blindly rely upon them; four levels of decision making, including involving an independent investigatory body, were utilized; Dr. Fuentes was afforded a due process hearing and Dr. Fuentes appealed and obtained an independent determination from Respondent's highest governing authority, its Board of Directors.

The Federal Investigator, after receiving the hospital response, communicated in writing to Alan Rogers:

In your EEOC charge, you allege you were subjected to discrimination based on your national origin when you were suspended from your job position.

The evidence collected does not indicate that your suspension was due to your national origin. Specifically, the Respondent provided information demonstrating that the suspension was based on grounds unrelated to your national origin. The Respondent noted that there was no record of your national origin or race in your personnel file. The Respondent became aware of your national origin only when the discrimination charge was filed, which mentioned your national origin and race. Prior to your suspension, no claims of discriminatory intent were raised during your hearing process. The grounds for your suspension were related to your conduct and communication with physicians and nurses. Moreover, during your Fair Hearing, the Respondent asserted that the complaints against you were unrelated to any claims of race or national origin. There is no evidence to suggest that your national origin was the actual reason for your Suspension.

> *Based on our review of the evidence, it is unlikely that additional investigation will result in a cause finding. However, if you have additional significant evidence that you believe supports your allegations, please submit it to me within 10 days of the date on this letter.*
>
> *If we do not hear from you, we may dismiss your case based on the available evidence. If your case is dismissed, EEOC will mail you a Dismissal and Notice of Rights, which will allow you to pursue your claims further by filing a private lawsuit within ninety (90) days of receipt of the Notice.*

Dr. Fuentes, advised by his lawyer, decided not to appeal the decision and let the Federal court dismiss the discrimination lawsuit.

After deliberation and several discussions with his lawyer, Dr. Fuentes filed a defamation lawsuit in the state of Arizona adding this lawsuit to the appeal against the hearing officer decision.

The Civil Lawsuit Outcome

The following weeks would have myriad witnesses contradicting each other. Each lawyer would try to convince the jury which version of events were reflective of the truth, until the jury was left to deliberate. But this time, the burden of proof was on behalf of Dr. Fuentes, with no hearsay admissible. In the absence of clear and tangible proof against Dr. Fuentes, the jury sided with Dr. Fuentes.

The filing foundation

The lawsuit filed was targeted to add to the appeal key persons who had defamed Dr. Fuentes and engaged in conspiracy

1. Nurse Simonar who defamed Dr. Fuentes in his claim by accusing him of (a) committing workplace violence, (b) "yelling" at Nurse Jane Clark, (c) committing a "verbal assault" against her, (d) creating a "hostile work environment."
2. Nurse Blevins defamed Dr. Fuentes in her complaint by (a) accusing him of creating a "hostile work environment," (b) "raised his voice in front of patients, and (c) "taking video of staff while patients are present."
3. Nurses Simonar and Blevins engaged in a civil conspiracy to damage Dr. Fuentes reputation, to secure the suspension and/or revocation of Dr. Fuentes' privileges, and to otherwise directly and indirectly cause him harm by each defaming and maligning him as detailed herein and coordinating with each other to procure statements from other nurses and others to be used against Dr. Fuentes.
4. The hospital defamed Dr. Fuentes through the statements made by human resources (Mrs. Clara Hariri and Alan Troy) to the MEC and the hearing officer.
5. The hospital conspired, through a scheme directed by the CEO and implemented in part by HR to defame him, mispresent facts about him, destroy evidence and conceal exculpatory information from the MEC to undermine his ability to retain his privileges, including by concealing the early availability of an assessment program and by coercively trying to have Dr. Fuentes waive his Fair Hearing rights under the hospital By-Laws.

6. Dr. Brauer and Dr. Balley defamed Dr. Fuentes through the statements they made during their testimony during the Fair Hearing. Indeed, the entire thoracotomy incident was extensively investigated, and Dr. Fuentes was never blamed or disciplined for causing any delay in Dr. Brauer performing the thoracotomy. The thoracotomy incident did not form any part of the MEC's Report that justified Dr. Fuentes suspension but was fabricated and brought during the hearing to create the illusion of a patient safety issue.
7. Dr. Fuentes has been damaged on account of this civil conspiracy including damage to his reputation, his medical practice, the suspension of his privileges, and the ongoing administrative and legal proceedings engendered thereby

By focusing on the defamation lawsuit against, Dr. Fuentes lawyer wanted to bring more power to the appeal at the court level, since any win in the defamation lawsuit will consequently impact the appeal process positively.

The First Day in Court

In a defamation lawsuit, the plaintiff, Dr. Fuentes, has the first opportunity to provide an overview of his case, explain the burden of proof, and argue how the evidence will demonstrate that his or her client has been defamed. The defendant, the hospital, then has an opportunity to provide an overview of their version of the events.

Two years after the "precautionary suspension of Dr. Fuentes" they were finally in court.

Dr. Fuentes lawyer started his opening statement in front of the Jury with the following words:

"A set up, an elaborated invention"

Ladies and Gentlemen of the jury, good morning, my name is Alan Rogers, I represent Dr. Fuentes. Within the next few days, we will demonstrate to this jury that this man (pointing at Dr. Fuentes), has been the victim of a set-up, a scheme to destroy his reputation and cover up major mistakes made by his hospital. Two years ago, a group of nurses unhappy with a turnover project which demonstrating their poor integrity, took advantage of spike event, during which Dr. Fuentes wasn't even the main actor, to conspire and create a narrative of a toxic physician, yelling, screaming and abusing his staff. These efforts should have failed, since an independent investigation cleared Dr. Fuentes, nevertheless under the pressure of nursing leadership, another investigation was launched by HR gathering exclusively people willing to trash Dr. Fuentes's character.

This allows HR to request Dr. Fuentes's precautionary suspension, which was granted based on lies. A week later, the medical executive committee met and took all information provided by HR as facts and decided to launch yet another investigation, the third one.

But this investigation was not aimed at finding the facts, but rather to justify and confirm retroactively the need to suspend Dr. Fuentes. That investigation took months and made sure to give more importance to negative testimonies, loosing positive testimonies and changing some statement made to vilify Dr. Fuentes, the most flagrant example was "Dr. Fuentes did not created an us versus them culture," became "he created an us versus them culture." The investigators sought testimonies from Dr. Fuentes's competitors, who saw this as an opportunity to finally get rid of him, to the point of fabulating clinical scenarios depicting him as an unsafe physician.

The medical executive committee split between the right thing to do, and political alliances decided to recommend a behavior assessment before bringing Dr. Fuentes back. For the jury clarification, behavior assessment can be requested at any time by the hospital leadership typically to assess the fitness of duty of a physician being rehabilitated after a psychiatrist, cognitive or physical condition. It was clear that Dr. Fuentes, at the peak of his career did not need a fitness for duty, but nevertheless agree to undergo that behavior assessment. A day before he officially registered, he received notification from the hospital lawyer that he needed to waive his hearing right before going to the assessment. It became clear to us that the hospital was trying to prevent him from taking any legal action in the future and make him admit that he was guilty from all accusations made. Not knowing what action, the MEC might take if he waived his right to a Fair Hearing, Dr. Fuentes chose not to waive his Hearing Rights and in fact challenged the MEC's decision to suspend his privileges in a Fair Hearing under the hospital By-Laws.

The By-Laws, however, contain a burden of proof that makes it virtually impossible for a physician to prevail at a "Fair Hearing," by requiring the physician to disprove by clear and convincing evidence the allegations against him, even if the allegations are based on hearsay.

A Hearing Officer, whose law firm performed services for the hospital and who rejected Dr. Fuentes's request to recuse himself presided over the Hearing and heard from 46 witnesses.

He acted as jury and judge during the process, even calling witnesses to support the hospital narrative and rejecting all testimonies on behalf of Dr. Fuentes. It was therefore not surprising that he found that Dr. Fuentes has not met his burden of proof and that the precautionary suspension was affirmed. He recommended that Dr. Fuentes be given the opportunity to attend the PRC program or any other appropriate assessment program so that the Hospital and its patients may regain his advanced skills and he is able to gain a more thorough understanding of and ability to control his interpersonal behavior. But Dr. Fuentes had already taken upon himself to go to the assessment performed by Vanderbilt in Nashville, in order to meet the MEC's recommendation, but this was rejected by the hospital since he didn't seek the board approval, but this approval would have been only possible by waiving his hearing right and accepting with guilt any outcome that pleases the hospital. Ladies and gentlemen, in summary Dr. Fuentes is a man of integrity who has been the victim of a large conspiracy; an advo-

> cate for his patients who for the past 2 years, exercised his right to protect himself and was not only coerced to waive this right but was denied any possibility to receive a fair hearing and appeal at the hospital level. This jury will be given an opportunity within the next few days to finally provide him justice.

Dick Kosakov, the hospital lawyer was next to start his opening statement.

It will be easy for the reader to imagine his speech, as he would be depicting Dr. Fuentes as the most disruptive physician.

The following weeks would have myriad witness contradicting each other. Each lawyer would try to convince the jury which version of events are reflective of the truth and the jury will be left to deliberate, but this time the burden of proof would be on behalf of Dr. Fuentes, hence his chance of prevailing would be much better.

In the real world, most of those cases get settled outside of court due to the inability of most physicians to sustain the cost associated with years of legal battles after months of struggle and torture at the hospital level. The legal system, by empowering hospitals to try and prosecute "disruptive physicians," has shifted the process and put them at the mercy of the hospital, whether they are truly problematic or not.

Dr. Fuentes's story is reflective of a much bigger problem, the inability of physicians to protect themselves from hospital and can only be resolve if all physicians are made aware of this troublesome "silent epidemy" upon us. It is only by lobbying together, and reaching out to law makers in Washington that the **Health Care Quality Improvement Act of 1986** can be amended to better protect physicians.

The Final Outcome: Top 5 Takeaways

1. Most cases involving actions against physicians get settled outside of court.
2. The financial burden associated with the legal cost put the physician in a disadvantageous position even in court.
3. The hospital always attempt to ruin financially the physician by delaying the process as much as possible.
4. Once in court, the burden of proof is on the side of the physician but time and money are on the side of the hospital.
5. The best chance to win the battle against the hospital is at the beginning of the case before the 30 days deadline.

CHAPTER 15

CONCLUSION

It has been three years since Dr. Fuentes was suspended and had his life turned upside down. However, his story isn't all tragic. At the end of these three years, he was able to rise from his struggles and was hired as a chief of interventional cardiology at a competing hospital in Phoenix, Arizona. With resilience, he was able to stand up to the hospital, exercise his right to a hearing, appeal at the hospital level, and take his case of defamation to the state courts.

In state court, the burden of proof was in his favor, with no hearsay admissible. Dr. Fuentes prevailed, as none of the witnesses who were so detrimental in the hospital hearings were credible in the absence of tangible evidence.

The suspension was voided, and he was retroactively fully reinstated.

For Dr. Fuentes, salvaging his career was not the only outcome of those three difficult years. He was able to emerge with new skills and a better understanding of optimal communication methods and healthy interpersonal interactions. Going forward, he will be able to recognize nuclear situations, and avoid any interactions that could escalate and lead to toxic confrontations.

Dr. Fuentes's resilience and application of his learned lessons will lead him to success in his new role. At the same time, his story becomes a lesson and a tale of caution for all practicing physicians.

Should we ever face such unjustified legal action from a large, powerful healthcare system that will do everything in its power to destroy a career, Dr. Fuentes shows us how a resilient physician can rise again and rediscover success.

www.ingramcontent.com/pod-product-compliance
Lightning Source LLC
LaVergne TN
LVHW090404210926
848480LV00002B/448
9798991785204